Glenn McGee

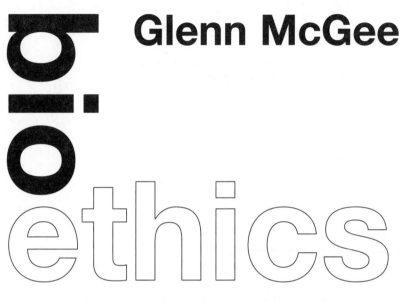

bio ethics

for beginners

*60 Cases and Cautions
from the Moral Frontier
of Healthcare*

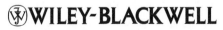

WILEY-BLACKWELL

A John Wiley & Sons, Ltd., Publication

This edition first published 2012
© 2012 John Wiley & Sons Inc.

Wiley-Blackwell is an imprint of John Wiley & Sons, formed by the merger of Wiley's
global Scientific, Technical and Medical business with Blackwell Publishing.

Registered Office
John Wiley & Sons Ltd, The Atrium, Southern Gate, Chichester, West Sussex,
PO19 8SQ, UK

Editorial Offices
350 Main Street, Malden, MA 02148-5020, USA
9600 Garsington Road, Oxford, OX4 2DQ, UK
The Atrium, Southern Gate, Chichester, West Sussex, PO19 8SQ, UK

For details of our global editorial offices, for customer services, and for information about how to
apply for permission to reuse the copyright material in this book please see our website at www
.wiley.com/wiley-blackwell.

The right of Glenn McGee to be identified as the author of the editorial material in this work has
been asserted in accordance with the UK Copyright, Designs and Patents Act 1988.

Library of Congress Cataloging-in-Publication Data

McGee, Glenn, 1967-
  Bioethics for beginners : 60 cases and cautions from the moral frontier of healthcare /
by Glenn McGee.
    p. cm.
  Includes bibliographical references and index.
  ISBN 978-0-470-65911-3 (hardback : alk. paper)
  1. Bioethics–Case studies. I. Title.
  QH332.M42 2012
  174–dc23

                                                                          2011044942

A catalogue record for this book is available from the British Library.

Set in 10/12.5 pt Plantin by Thomson Digital, Noida, India
Printed in Singapore by Ho Printing Singapore Pte Ltd

1   2012

bio
ethics
for beginners

For Summer

Contents

Caution 4 Reproduce at Your Own Peril 40

Caution 5 Don't Sweat the Nano-Sized Stuff 57

Caution 6 The State Will Protect Your Health Right Up Until It Doesn't 69

Caution 7 "Do No Harm" Has Become "Care for Yourself" 86

Contents

Preface

The Chief of Bioethics

A Bioethicist is not a sheriff. That's a good thing.

My children have no idea what I do. According to my eleven-year-old, bioethics is not a job, it's where I am before I come home and what I do on my computer. That I am editor of a medical journal means little to him, because he is quite sure that this means that I spend a bunch of time writing a magazine with no pictures. When I describe research about parenthood, or genetics, in what I assume to be eleven-year-old speak, he looks at me as though I must be avoiding the grading of papers, what real teachers do. My nine-year-old is more pragmatic: "What did you do today, Daddy?" Well, I wrote a bunch of emails, talked to a bunch of people, and stared at a legal brief designed to preserve patents on genetic information. "Oh, so you sat around. Why didn't you just come home?" They've heard of bioethics, and they hear Daddy talk on the radio or see him on TV. But it sounds just like the talk on the phone. My father was a professor, and I knew what he did. He taught and graded papers. The sole evidence, to my kids, that I do a job is that I have had badges. Various ones, tossed on tables, from conferences. But one in particular, issued to me in 2005 by New York State's public health labs, is the kicker: it identified me as "Chief" of the labs' Office of Bioethics. When he saw it, my son patted me on the back for finding a real job: he thought I was a police chief. I must have been protecting someone.

The point of this story, or at least *my* point, isn't this father's instinctive need for the respect of his sons. It is that my sons are not all that different from the rest of biomedical science and society. After forty years, bioethics is still an enigma to the NPR-listening crowd, and all-too-often revered by the "public" only when it purveys ideology or polices misconduct. The research that we do, the cases on which we consult, the changes in healthcare that have come from involving the people who are sometimes called bioethicists, are lost to almost everyone but the few academics, media, and policy wonks who read our work or participate in our consultations or ask us to work with them on a project with ethical implications. And that is a problem. Most of the broadly read articles about bioethics, some authored by ethicists themselves, have castigated bioethicists for being too heavily indebted to industry, or for being irrelevant, or for refusing to take stands in a coherent way, even about our own standards for good practice in our field. Bioethics has become one of, if not the, fastest growing academic disciplines, and there are more students aspiring to work in the field than one could ever have dreamt. But the role of the people who work in the field is incomprehensible to most unless it is framed as "fireman" or "professor."

Success is sometimes a curse. The presence of bioethics in virtually every major debate about social values has made it more difficult to explain why bioethicists, whomever we are, cannot explain what it is that we actually do, how to recognize when we are doing it well, or that there is a difference between providing expertise about ethical issues and being a moral superhero. How can any scholarly field be broad enough to address – indeed, be at the center of – debates over Terri Schiavo, stem cell research, the rationing of drugs for a pandemic or respirators after a hurricane, the risks of clinical research, the sale of human organs, the creation of artificial life, and the role of physicians in torture?

In the forty years since American biochemist, Van Rensselaer Potter, it would seem, coined the term, interest in bioethics has spawned hundreds of institutes, more than a dozen journals, and many degree-granting university programs. But neither bioethics' practice nor those styled as practitioners are defined in the same way by any dozen people outside academia. Even academics are split on whether bioethics is in exile from philosophy departments or a subspecialty of medicine or something else altogether. Colleagues, bosses, students, community groups, and potential donors ask whether bioethics involves real scholarship and teaching, or if it is merely a shill for regulatory, corporate, or political interests. Even those of us who work in the field are divided on whether bioethics is a discipline, whether we should have certification (badges, anyone?), and whether there is the need for a code of ethics for ethicists, as though those who work in bioethics are not content experts but rather ethical "superheros" whose own moral lives are the measure of their ability to teach. We don't even discuss that for members of the faculty of departments of religion, though, the annual meeting of the American Academy of Religion and of the Society for Christian Ethics, have been described as having the character of frat parties. A colleague of mine once said that academics who work in ethics across the field, in fact, typically choose as their area of expertise, however unconscious the choice, that area of study that least corresponds with the mores that guide their own life: the man who studies the ethics of character has none, the woman who writes about empathy could care less about those around her. Society knows just enough about ethics to trade in the silly supposition that the study of an area presupposes a superhuman moral life. I certainly hope that isn't a fair standard, because I for one am a *human* scholar.

There are as many ways to parse the jobs and activities of bioethicists as there are problems under study in the field. Many use the title to describe or advertise their work. Those who write in the peer-reviewed journals of bioethics, teach and work in institutes devoted to the subject, and are members of the key organizations, clearly qualify for the appellation. Scholars in bioethics now have a huge impact on science and medical policy, and those who pretend to be bioethicists in order to put that mantle on their political or religious arguments, do so precisely because they recognize the increasing importance of the field.

At a time, however, when political columnists, fundamentalist zealots, and untrained aficionados not only call themselves bioethicists but also are eligible to work on a presidential commission on the subject, many of those who should be calling themselves bioethicists in virtue of their training and scholarship instead repudiate that label. Though tempting, it would be a mistake to recoil in horror as bioethics becomes politicized. A good sign of the health of bioethics, in fact, is the healthy debate and political action elicited by bioethics scholarship. It would be bad news indeed for the future of debate about ethics in medicine and science if no one cared about the controversial conclusions reached by those who study and write in the area. And that bioethicists engage in politicization of their field seems understandable as well – as long as it is clear that they do it off the clock.

I'll admit, there's a certain allure to the idea of a job that my child can understand. But I know there is something that they definitely understand: rules. Rules define the moral scope of the world in which we live, they guide our thoughts and actions, they prescribe the limits of how we should interact with our peers, patients, and the public. Without rules, we would live in anarchy and without consequences for ignoring those rules, we would be left to act on our most base and opportunistic impulses.

My "chief of bioethics" badge really is an artifact of a time when bioethics had to be explained not only to children but also to funding agencies, the media, and policymakers. We no longer live in that time. Today most leaders in science and medicine know that bioethics, properly understood, isn't a police force, a task force, or the product of a president's commission.

But it is about providing guidance, when needed but not always when invited, to those at the cutting edges of science and medicine. Giving them the green light (morally speaking), noting when proceed with caution, or reminding them that speed can be deadly. Bioethicists are an elitist, powermongering, or advocacy-based group, but instead we depend on a symbiotic relationship between researchers, practitioners, policymakers, and the public. And out of that relationship we strive to make the outcome of our collaborator's work more justifiable, reasonable, and fair.

All appearances to the contrary, the explosion of interest in bioethics and even the groping to be called a bioethicist represent a recognition that the field of bioethics is coming of age. As are my children, all of whom – even the 17-year-old – understand the value and importance of rules, even if they rarely follow them.

This book, too, chronicles the missteps and the successes of some of medicine and science most important events in the last decade and from these articulates the "new rules" for ethical science and medicine in the twenty-first century.

Acknowledgements

This book is the result in large part of the editorial, advisory, and audience response input of dozens of people in science and medicine, including those who attended countless lectures and those who have been forced to edit the essays herein for publication. Equally, a team of my very generous peers participated in congealing from a variety of my activities in translational medicine what I hope is a coherent and underlying thesis: that at the beginning of the era of highly mixed, personalized genomic medicine, when we no longer know how to describe creation or death and our powers have increased almost as fast as those of our computers, wisdom will come not from "intuitive fear" of the future but from a pragmatic look at the past and at the goals inherent to our human natures.

Actively involved in the preparation of the manuscript, among others, were co-authors of some of my work, Arthur Caplan PhD and Summer Johnson McGee PhD.

Researchers and editors included Kelly Hills, Jessica Stanley, and Miriam Aziz.

David Magnus PhD provided assistance both as co-editor of the *American Journal of Bioethics* and thus on numerous editorial materials produced for that venue and also as a close friend and close reader when called upon.

This book would never have happened but for the generous contributions of the Francis Foundation and the John B. Francis Chair in Bioethics at my scholarly home, the unique Center for Practical Bioethics and the assistance and guidance of my colleagues there including Myra Christopher, President.

Caution One

Tip-Toe When Walking on the Bleeding Edge

Case 1   The Dangers of Creating Life in the Lab

Synthetic biology is receiving much attention in the media and in churches, schools and offices around the world. The issue is the creation of life in the laboratory. And the reactions range from excitement to ethical outrage to horror at the new potential for bioterrorism.

First, the scientists at The Institute for Genomic Research (TIGR) in Rockville, Md., published the details of their effort to isolate the minimum number of genes an organism needs to survive in *Science*. They reported on a project in which they aim to create a kind of life form by building each bit of the genetic code for a type of simple bacterium called mycoplasma in the laboratory, then stacking the bits together like toy blocks. At the end of the effort, the scientists can prove not only that the bits of genetic information they stack together can be artificially "animated" into acting just like any other bacterium, but also that the most important parts of bacteria and viruses can be synthesized at will in a laboratory.

But to build a virus with a minimum complement of genes that would allow it to perform the same tasks is not the same as making a more complex organism, even an amoeba. Let alone one that can self-replicate. That is what Craig Venter did.

Craig Venter set the scientific, religious, and political worlds on fire when he announced that he had created a new organism by synthesizing DNA from one bacteria and inserting it into another. This time the organism included not only the minimal number of genes for survival,

Bioethics for Beginners: 60 Cases and Cautions from the Moral Frontier of Healthcare, First Edition. Glenn McGee.
© 2012 John Wiley & Sons, Ltd. Published 2012 by John Wiley & Sons, Ltd.

but also those required for self-replication. In doing so he created the first self-replicating synthetic bacteria.

And as a result of his research, even President Obama has been paid close attention to synthetic biology. Hijacking his own Presidential Commission's agenda, he asked that group to report within 6 months about the ethical, social, and legal implications of Craig Venter's research. That group concluded that "prudent vigilance" – a combination of Aristotelian notions of prudence combined with a eviscerated precautionary principle – is the approach that will allow science to flourish without running amok.

But in one sense there is a prior step: simply understanding what the current state of science can and cannot do. The creation of a self-replicating synthetic cell, while important scientifically, was not "playing God" or rearranging the natural order. Upon reflection, nearly every religious group – from the Vatican to Talmudic scholars – has come out in favor of the use of synthetic biology for its multitude of practical applications. In Venter's case, he has argued that this technology would allow for using synthetic cells to create biofuels, and ultimately mitigating the effects of climate change.

And while there are legitimate concerns about the more unseemly sides of synthetic biology, building in protections to prevent those misuses of the technology while allowing science to flourish has been the magic sweet spot that regulators and policy makers have been trying to find.

Outbreaks via e-mail?

The possible implications of synthetic biology can be downright terrifying. In little vials we see in movies like *Outbreak*, a few tiny bits of the most deadly viruses of our time are stored for research. Behind steel doors, frozen, with mighty ventilation and filtration systems, bits of anthrax, smallpox and countless biological variants of these viruses are kept for analysis at the US Centers for Disease Control and Prevention.

I'm really glad they sit there behind lock and key, and I bet you share my fear that the repository of viruses in the former Soviet Union is sometimes imperiled by fighting and political turmoil. Lots of folks would just as soon see our last bits of deadly virus eliminated.

Guess what? The synthetic biology research opens the door to a whole new problem: viral hacking. Who needs to find a tiny sample of smallpox, when you can synthesize it from scratch on a $1,000 iMac connected to a $10,000 gene synthesizer? If viruses can be manipulated and created, their

2

genetic codes can also be e-mailed around the world and built from innocuous lab materials using the same technology.

For ethicists and society, the puzzle is to identify how scientists should proceed, and for what reasons they might have to slow down. But this is not always an easy proposition.

And in some cases, ethicists are not the right people to puzzle about the problem. The problems of dual-use, the problem that scientific advances and new technologies, like synthetic biology, can be used for both good and bad outcomes is a problem that must include public health experts, national security consultants, experts in international law, scientists, and others. Synthetic biology opens a whole new world of biological terrorism *and* environmental restoration. We will have to think fast to stay ahead of the power synthetic biology puts in the hands of scientists and terrorists. There is reason to be cautious indeed.

Case 2   Design: More Intelligent Every Day

Thanks to a 2005 court decision, children in Kansas now learn that the fossil record of our planet holds evidence of "irreducibly complex" traits, biological wonders that seem too sophisticated to be products of natural selection. Advocates of intelligent design argue that such complexity of biological life reveals evidence of a designer.

A different sort of designer is working in the nascent filed of synthetic biology. These scientists generate novel biological functions through the design and construction of living systems. Synthetic biologists manipulate the most complex biological interactions using the tools of engineering and computer science. It has borne fruit in the design of genomes, proteins, devices, integrated biological systems, and even cell-circuit hybrids. Synthetic biologists use evolution as a method. That seems pretty intelligent.

William Paley probably wasn't imagining such researchers when he expounded on the form of the intelligent design theory that children will be learning in Kansas. In his publication in 1800, *Natural Theology*, in which he was the first to suggest the idea, he wrote that just as a watch requires a watchmaker, the unexplainable complexities of nature can only be explained by the work of an intelligent creator. A small army of contemporary disciples has advanced the claim that for a variety of reasons intelligent design is a necessary antecedent to the teaching of evolution in schools.

Intelligent design theory might well be inspirational to those in synthetic biology, whose job it is to use their own brains to make imaginative sue of the raw materials and processes of creation. But the feeling would not be mutual. The Kansas school board spoke of its fear of evolutionists playing God. To an intelligent design proponent, synthetic biology is the blasphemous use of God's erector set. If biology is the story of the sacrosanct plan of an omniscient being, rather than the vicissitudes of natural selection, humans have a hard time explaining why they are tinkering with the works.

According to a February 2011 Gallup poll only 40 percent of the US population believes in evolution. Of the 25 percent who say they absolutely reject the theory, it is many of these citizens who have gone to court and to the polls to push the ideas that intelligent design is an important scientific theory.

They do so with religious zeal. A thousand miles away from Kansas in Dover, Pa., families who fired a school board that had insisted on teaching intelligent design are now in grave danger of incurring the wrath of God, according to televangelist Pat Robertson. "If you stick your finger in God's eye too many times, maybe you should try praying to Darwin when the next disaster strikes."

Some people working in synthetic biology wouldn't mind sticking a finger in Pat Robertson's eye. A leading synthetic biologist once said to me that she is working so hard on building and animating an artificial bacterium primarily so that she can prove to advocates of intelligent design that it doesn't take a God to create life. I wish her luck, and Godspeed.

The real worry, though, is about the future of science. Children educated in a system in which untestable statements of faith are treated as privileged hypotheses are hardly prepared to face a world in which evolution is a fact of life. The next generation of scientists will face the rapid evolution of viruses and the implications of decreasing diversity in animals. We cannot afford to raise a generation of doctors who believe that drug-resistant bacteria are a punishment from God rather than an evolutionary process induced by the misuse of antibiotics. Whomever or whatever created the universe, let's hope they wanted us to be intelligent, too.

Case 3   "Shroom" Science: Safe and Effective?

Are Ritalin and psilocybin equivalent in terms of effect and safety?

In the August 2006 issue of *Psychopharmacology*, Johns Hopkins researchers published a study in which some subjects were given psilocybin and then asked to relate their experiences. Francisco Moreno of the University of Arizona published in the November 2006 issue of the *Journal of Clinical Psychiatry* his patients' reports that psilocybin helped them with migraine headaches. Harbor-UCLA Medical Center psychiatrist Charles Grob told the *Chronicle of Higher Education* that he is giving the compound to patients dying of cancer to see whether it eases pain by relieving anxiety.

The study of so-called magic mushrooms isn't new; it could be argued that it is celebrating its 55th anniversary this year. It began, as best anyone can tell, when Wall Street banker R. Gordon Wasson documented his trip to a healer in Oaxaca, Mexico, whose brew, he claimed, enabled him to see the reality of ideas and concepts. His 1957 essay in *Life* magazine excited the imaginations of scientists around the world. Sandoz patented the two active chemicals in the mushrooms, calling the compounds psilocin and psilocybin. Chaos ensued as researchers struggled to do excellent scientific work using a family of substances whose effects – to put it mildly – were not easily measurable using the tools of the time.

The scientists who used psilocybin in their research in the 1960s poked at the nature of consciousness, but this particular compound just refused to be caged by ordinary scientific conventions. Paper after paper stabbed at descriptions of the effects and utility of psilocybin, but scalar measures of transcendence just could not capture its effects, or side effects. A few of the leading scientists engaged in its study, most notoriously Harvard psychologist Timothy Leary, simply abandoned the strictures of scientific research as insufficient to grasp the power of psilocybin.

By the time the FDA banned hallucinogenic drugs in 1970, the majority of those experimenting with mushrooms were not in universities. Hallucinogens became part of a counterculture that aged quickly. By the 1980s, the next counterculture devoted to brain modification was moving in a completely different direction, experimenting with highly addictive stimulants, such as cocaine, which assist in thinking faster, concentrating harder, and intensifying ordinary experiences.

Time passes, and what's old becomes new again. In 2007 millions of people took legal stimulants and antidepressants. A decades-long quest for endless work capacity, unfettered concentration, and happiness on-demand has perhaps hastened the return of those who wonder whether the touch of transcendence could provide new insights into treating the maladies that have become rampant in our time. And indeed, new studies suggest that psilocybin may offer hope in treating a few of them, ranging from obsessive-compulsive disorder to rampant addiction.

With the dramatically enhanced ability of neural imaging to identify changes in brain state, and advances in the genetics of neuroscience, it is no wonder that some of those who researched psilocybin in the 1970s have begun to point again to the potential of that compound. Magic mushrooms are not addictive and have been around more than half a century. So should we really be worried about the potential that new research will lead a new generation to "turn on, tune in, and drop out"? Yes.

Ethics committees examining the research programs underway with hallucinogens need to be mindful that what sparked the widespread illegal use of psilocybin in the 1970s was not its mystical power but the reports of its safety and efficacy coming out of the leading institutions of higher learning in the United States. Scientists are acting with great care this time around, but let's avoid a bad trip.

Hallucinogens have not been scientifically demonstrated to be either safe or effective enough to be used in the treatment of any disease. Studies of them should be undertaken only when investigators avoid sending subtle messages about the safety or delight of chewing on backyard mushrooms. For example, in the Hopkins study subjects were given either Ritalin or psilocybin, sending the terribly premature message that the two substances are in any sense equivalent in terms of effect or safety. It would have been much better to compare psilocybin with, well, anything other than a compound prescribed to tens of millions and often abused by those seeking better cognition.

Thankfully that study was all but ignored by the media. When it comes to hallucinogens, if the research sends the wrong message, drop it. Or rather, don't.

Case 4   A Robot Code of Ethics

Should we require robot makers to program in a code of ethics?

The South Korean people really love robots. Industry in South Korea receives millions in government subsidies to develop them. Park Hye-Young, of the South Korean Ministry of Commerce, Industry, and Energy's robot team, said in a statement to the French Press Agency that the Ministry hoped "to have a robot in every South Korean household between 2015 and 2020," and predicted that these robots would develop "strong intelligence." South Koreans are not the only ones embracing robots. Already iRobot, a company founded by Rodney Brooks, director of the MIT Artificial Intelligence Lab, has sold 6 million Roombas, a little robotic vacuum cleaner. The promise of the robot vacuum and its cousins is that the home robot will become faster, more reliable, and more cost-effective than human domestic work. It has to get this "strong intelligence" part down first. My Roomba is a one-trick pony, sucking dirt while rolling in circles and slapping into the same walls every day as it relearns a 12 in × 12 in room. This is not Rosie from *The Jetsons*. But the more important issue regarding today's domestic robots and the future is not so much about intelligence as it is about ethics. If you ever watched the Roomba-sized robots hack each other to bits on the aptly named BBC-5 television program, *Robot Wars*, you know the fear that lives in the souls of many who will never buy a domestic robot: that their Roomba would one day awaken like the robots of *The Terminator*. A robot with sinister intentions, without ethics, or adhering dispassionately to a code of ethics where intuition and subtlety is required (remember *RoboCop*?) has been the fuel of science fiction for decades. Should we require robot makers to program in a code of ethics to domestic products?

Perhaps robots should be afraid of us too; whether or not they dream of electric sheep, the robotic sex toys under development are purveyed as better-than-real-life companions. But they are plastic and metal, not human. As humans build robots that learn what their owners desire, the dilemma of the robots of *Blade Runner* emerges: What do humans owe "purpose-built" machines who begin to reach awareness, or to so resemble awareness that it becomes a selling point? Should laws be written to protect robots from us, by requiring robot makers to stop short of, say, robosexual devices that learn to be incredibly intimate with humans and yet are owed nothing? If so, do we create such laws in the interest of robots, or to preserve our own human dignity by choosing not to create a new kind of slave, whether or not that slave is fully aware?

The South Korean government has taken a progressively minded step by convening a committee to draw up an ethical code to prevent humans from abusing robots and vice versa. The code draws in part on the work of science-fiction writer Isaac Asimov, and specifically, according to Park, on the three laws Asimov proposed for robot ethics in a 1942 story, "Runaround." They are: (1) A robot may not injure a human being or, through inaction, allow a human being to come to harm; (2) A robot must obey orders given it by human beings, except where such orders would conflict with the first law; and (3) A robot must protect its own existence as long as such protection does not conflict with the first or second law.

7

Likewise, a committee of EURON, the European Robotics Research Network, met in Genoa, Italy, in June, 2006 and concluded that a code must be created to deal with the problems of hostility to and from robots, as well as how to avoid accidents, trace robots, ensure the secrecy of their data, and monitor the nature of their intelligence, which one member of the latter commission aptly described as "intelligence of an alien sort."

It remains to be seen whether robots will become in some sense intelligent androids, capable of interacting as peers with humans and other parts of the world. In the meantime, we are much closer to making robots with "strong intelligence" than we are to creating a code of ethics to guide our stewardship of tin men, or to protecting humanity from misbegotten robotics. Either the effort to create a code of ethics to shape the evolution of robotics will be embraced, or we may reap the consequences.

It only remains to be seen who will wake up first.

Case 5   No More Periods, Period

For decades, fertility research has successfully decoupled sex from reproduction, forever altering women's position and power in the developed world. Among all methods of contraception, none is as well known or influential as "the pill." Now, its power has been kicked up a notch, and the pill is poised to do what some say will disrupt the very nature of the XX sex. This leaves us with one question: In the next step of the evolution of women's contraception, should we eliminate the last major physical manifestation of the reproductive cycle, menstruation?

The birth control pill contains hormones that stop the release of an egg, which in turn prevents the buildup of the uterine lining. Bleeding occurs on traditional oral birth control (21 days of hormone pills, 7 days of placebo) only because of the interruption of the hormones during placebo days. A newer oral contraceptive, Seasonale, reduces the period still further, with only seven placebo days every three months. But the newest, continuous low-dose contraceptive, Lybrel, stops the period entirely.

No one disputes that eliminating menstruation could free women from a variety of uncomfortable or even dangerous symptoms, from severe pain and cramping to emotional swings. For some, these symptoms have a profound impact, but not necessarily one viewed as cause to eliminate periods altogether, until recently. Now, the message is clear and direct to the consumer: In the twenty-first century, women who are not seeking pregnancy need not waste time and energy with menstruation.

What happens to human nature if the period comes to an end? In one example, Canadian researcher Christine Hitchcock told the *New York Times* she worries about products that "turn your body on and off like a tap." Her concern was, in part, about the unknown consequences of stopping menstruation entirely, a concern shared by others who have asked whether the long-term side effects of such medication can really be predicted to any reliable degree. Other opponents of the end of the period argue vociferously that doing so is unnatural. Menstruation is not a "sickness," they say – it gives woman a sense of identity, and eliminating menstruation in a mammal that does not show estrus will profoundly alter the very nature of human nature.

Paradoxically, the concept of "what's natural" is one that supporters also use to justify the new contraceptives. On the Seasonale web site, Patricia Sulak, professor of obstetrics and gynecology at the Texas A&M University System Health Science Center – College of Medicine, argues that it's not natural to have as many periods as modern women do, since previous generations had more children and breastfed longer. "Today we're having hundreds of periods in our lifetime, whereas a century ago we were only having a few periods. One might say that that's not natural; that's not what we were designed to do."

But these are preposterous arguments. The question is not whether stopping menstruation is natural. The question is: Is it safe? Menstruation isn't what defines a woman, since women are still women after meno-pause, and menstruating women often live with ailments that stop their periods. Menstruation is something that happens to women, just like sweating and headaches; consequently, arguing that no-period contra-ceptives alter human nature is no different than saying the same about antiperspirants or analgesics.

It is a stretch to suggest that menstruation will be considered a disease, and it certainly makes sense to conduct research aimed at improving women's quality of life. One could also note the billions of dollars spent on feminine hygiene products that serve no procreative purpose, or the environmental consequences of making and disposing of billions of pads and tampons. The real issue here is women's right to make choices about their reproductive systems and sexuality, and even about what risks they are willing to take with either, just as when the FDA first approved the pill in 1960. Period.

Case 6 Search Me, Shape Me, Any Way You Want Me

In his April 2006 column, Jack Woodall suggested that we bring the "don't be evil" technology of Google to the rapidly advancing field of brain-computer interfacing. It'd be dandy, he argued, to order the information in our brains in hierarchical fashion. In short, he wants to Google the brain.

But the more compelling argument, to me, is that a search engine-style filter would do for the brain what it does for academic research – find the good stuff fast. It's a beautiful dream and it will probably come true within my lifetime. And as long as my brain doesn't gain banner ads, spy ware, or pop-up windows, I'd probably sign up for the Woodall experiment.

Remembering is everything in the New World. Everything you have ever written can be stored: every e-mail, grant, paper, Power Point presentation, syllabus, recommendation letter, list of plans, and perhaps even your bad poetry and divorce decree. And if it can be stored, it can be accessed, filtered, and searched.

John Dewey, the philosopher most responsible for the development of the social sciences, wrote a large amount – by one estimation more than 13,000 pages of manuscript and perhaps a gigabyte of searchable correspondence. Historians of science in twenty years will find that even "B-list" scholars of today produce ten times that volume of information in the course of a decade, not including the vault of other people's data we store in case we need it.

My most disorganized friends, or at least the smart ones, are steadily working their way toward scanning all the paper in their offices onto hard drives, turning piles of nomenclature and unfinished projects into a different kind of pile. Desks get cleaned, computers get filled. But the clutter is still there, it's just hidden more effectively. Those who scan their worlds without clearing out the junk and learning to sort information just make their messes more intimate. I don't need to remember a lot of what is stored around my office or in the corners of my mind.

There is something to be said for forgetting. Nietzsche argued that those who cannot forget are quickly driven to madness. The ultimate stoic, Epictetus, implored Roman soldiers to kiss everyone in their lives goodbye every time they walked out the door, pointing to the importance of focusing on the present. Beta-blockers such as Inderal can literally disconnect memories from their emotional impact; predictably, many victims of trauma are eager to kill the pain that data stored in the brain can cause.

10

Numerous studies on the most stressful activities in human life moving, divorce, and the death of a parent or child – suggest that the stress of a life change is mostly a matter of cognitive dissonance, the pain of remembering what is lost. Santayana, famous for his statement that those who forget the past are doomed to repeat it, wrote nonetheless: "I would I might forget that I am I, and break the heavy chain that binds me fast."

The problem with hooking search engine technology up to my mind is that part of my identity, which I happen to like, has to do with my ability to really forget, to shape my own life. Perhaps a search engine could make that easier, perhaps I could block out things that are awful. But then again, Kierkegaard wrote: "Marry, and you will regret it. Do not marry, and you will also regret it." And he didn't even have a good memory.

Today's search engine is no better than the myopic man behind the algorythmic curtain, and I am not sure what he'd make of the detritus in my brain.

Brains are great. Machines are great. Connecting them is great. But before the interface becomes my identity, I'd like it to be just a bit more refined.

Case 7   A Bloody Mess

From the moment of trauma, whether for wounded soldiers, victims of motor vehicle accidents, or children hit by bullets, the best solution to blood loss is, obviously, blood. But many ambulances don't carry blood because it is extremely volatile. Paramedics can offer saline solution, sometimes even laced with nonblood "expanders," but saline can't ferry oxygen around the bloodstream to keep cells alive.

Enter Polyheme, an oxygen-carrying blood substitute that promised to revolutionize emergency medicine. Polyheme is made from a modified hemoglobin molecule, and it carries oxygen. It is more resilient than blood, with a much longer shelf life and better tolerance of the conditions at the scene of a trauma and in transport. It does not need to be matched to a patient's blood type. And as a bonus, unlike an organ transplant or blood transfusion, there is no risk that a communicable disease will be passed in the process.

Oxygen-carrying blood substitutes have been tried for years on consenting research subjects with mixed results, but enough hope has existed that since 1970, no fewer than three companies have fixed their sights on

11

making one. Polyheme's sponsor and manufacturer, Northfield Labs, sought approval for use on the battlefield or in a trauma helicopter near you. So with what could amount to a significant advance for trauma medicine being on the brink of approval, why were the airwaves, newspapers, academic journals, and magazines riddled with stories about whether research subjects in the trial are human guinea pigs?

The answer is that communities where this research has begun have been caught off guard. In Phase I and Phase II trials of Polyheme, all subjects were required to give informed consent. Eventually, Polyheme had to be tried on typical patients who would benefit from artificial blood: victims of trauma. Of course, the vast majority of trauma victims cannot give informed consent. Thus, regulations passed in the mid-1990s called the Final Rule allow such research, provided a list of precautions is followed, including something called "community consultation." The idea is that while enrollees would be too ill to consent, investigators would have informed the community about the trial in advance; anyone who doesn't want to participate can prospectively opt-out by, for example, wearing an armband.

The best laid plans

After Northfield Lab's researchers informed the community about Polyheme, emergency medical technicians were to randomly administer either saline solution or Polyheme to trauma patients who are in hemorrhagic shock. The control group receives blood, the standard of care. Those randomized to Polyheme receive it for no more than 12 hours; part of that time may be in the hospital when they would otherwise be given blood.

The problem was that most people in the communities where Polyheme trials were going on, from Illinois to North Carolina to New York, didn't seem to know a bit about it. Emergency medical research is a bloody mess right now because Polyheme, once unknown to potential subjects, suddenly came onto the public radar, but only because of concerns that include undisclosed or inappropriate risks to subjects in the in-hospital phase of the study, worries about whether the sponsor has withheld data from investigators, and criticisms from organizations such as the Senate Appropriations Committee and consumer advocacy groups.

It has become clear that patients worry about emergency research and that new methods for informing the community must be devised and tested before proceeding with trials that have such potential to destroy public trust in research. We know some scientific facts: Saline solution doesn't carry oxygen. Polyheme does. Therein lies the potential for a miracle. Polyheme, and other substances like it, are certain to end up on the Congressional black list because communities that do not trust researchers are not going to let them ride in ambulances.

Northfield goes on record about PolyHeme

You'd think that Northfield Labs (the sponsor/owner of PolyHeme) would have something thoughtful to say about how that company, in the middle of a tornado, will be dealing with the matter.

Nope. No committee, no ethics team, no refinement of materials, and still no answers of consequence to the charge that there was a cover up of material that should have been published. No comment of consequence even when the Johns Hopkins researcher the company had said would clear everything up was subsequently denied the data he needed to give that speech.

You'd think Northfield would want, in the face of all this controversy, to resolve any doubts that might otherwise need to be shared with the community. But instead the company seemed to have a zero ethics plan:

"Is this a good reg? Is it perfect? Can it be better? Can it be worse? Those are important policy questions that we feel we can and should address," said Steven Gould, chief executive of Northfield Laboratories, the firm that makes and is studying PolyHeme. "To do research without prospective informed consent defies what we would all say is good ethical practices, so you have this conundrum."

Yes. So you will be doing what? Asked by the *American Journal of Bioethics* to respond to an article written about the Polyheme trials, Northfield refused. Asked to participate in a discussion with principal investigators of the trial about how to refine community consultation so that communities can understand the ongoing issues that are in articles like this one, the company offered to consider the idea then didn't reply. Asked whether they would like to try to convene an ethics review, board, study or to participate in any other review of the associated issues with others, there was no reply.

The conundrum was there, no question. But it wasn't about the ethics of research without informed consent, or about failure to respond adequately (in the minds of many) to charges that their study was designed so that it intentionally requires that subjects receive Polyheme instead of blood even after they arrive in hospitals (and without consent), contrary to the standard of care.

No, the conundrum was how Northfield managed to avoid killing off resuscitation research entirely, while sitting in wait for a Senator who is mad as hops. Fortunately, the Polyheme trials were entirely stopped and Northfield disappeared from the research ethics radar screen. Doing significant damage to emergency research for years, the Polyheme study taught us that research regulations are there for a reason and failure to adhere to them can create one bloody mess indeed.

Case 8   Stem Cells: The Goo of Life and the Debate of the Century

Everyone is up in arms about stem cell research: adult versus embryonic, iPSCs, and parthenotes. And maybe not up in arms exactly. But certainly everyone has a champion, a favorite kind of stem cell, the cell on the verge of curing cancer, macular degeneration, or male pattern baldness.

But don't believe the hype

Pluripotent stem cell research has the potential to revolutionize medicine, pluripotent cells seem to be the "goo of life," a cellular biological discovery (by James Thompson and JohnGearhardt) as revolutionary as the spiraling of DNA identified in 1953 by molecular biology pioneers James Watson and Francis Crick.

Once derived from an early-stage embryo, they may be directed to grow into virtually any kind of cell line. Liver cells, brain cells, bone cells, skin cells: If you need cells or tissue, we may soon be able to grow compatible, stem cell-derived cell lines to help.

But as we have now learned, pluripotent stem cells can be developed from more than just embryos. Induced pluripotent stem cells (iPSCs) uses a technique whereby pluripotent stem cells are created artificially from adult somatic cells. By using the correct growth factors and hormones, "the goo" transforms from adult skin cells, for example, to pluripotent cells with specific gene expression.

Then there is the so called "adult stem cell" camp, those who herald mesochymal stem cells as the solution to all that ails the world. These multipotent stem cells have been successfully used to differentiate into bone, cartilage, fat, and pancreatic cells. The relative advantage of these cells is, of course, once harvested from the human body and amplified, they can be injected right back into the patients they came from without any need to change the cell's potency.

Many could benefit

A few of the diseases for which stem cells, whether embryonic, iPSC, or mesenchymal, might offer therapies or cures: Parkinson's disease, Alzheimer's disease, diabetes, heart disease, stroke, arthritis, birth defects, osteoporosis, spinal cord injuries, and burns made the list, as well as most cancers. That accounts for more than half of all Americans, and Patient's Cure estimates that 148 million Americans will be candidates for stem cell therapy. That is once stem cells can be used as therapies.

On the other hand, you could scarcely imagine a more controversial field of research. While opinion polls suggest that the majority of Americans support the use of very early embryonic cells for this research, most Americans are both vehemently opposed to abortion and frightened to death by what they hear about a few outlying infertility clinics and practices in the United States.

Catholic bioethicist Richard Dorflinger has argued that embryos should not be used under any circumstances, even if the embryo is discarded in freezers at fertility clinics. It is difficult to imagine, other pro-life groups have argued, a bigger destruction of human life than that entailed by a massive stem cell research campaign.

Existing Federal law (the Dickey–Wicker Amendment) prohibits the destruction of embryos for research, but NIH has made a distinction between the destruction of embryos, which the agency cannot fund, and research on resultant stem cell lines, which it can. Pro-life scholars counter that federal funding of pluripotent stem cell research is the same as funding abortions.

The abortion debate is certainly one of the greatest failures of American democracy to empower and civilize public discourse. Lives are lost, careers and esteem destroyed, and religion made to serve as a political football.

We have needed to separate stem cell research from the abortion debate for more than a decade and we still keep failing to do so. The creation of iPSCs and advances with mesenchymal stem cells can help skirt some of these debates, but they do nothing to resolve them and do little to differentiate how people think about "stem cell research" writ large. The critical issues here are tough, and they require us all to do some deep thinking about how we want to understand human life and dignity and about how we want our social institutions to work.

The issues

First, what is an embryo? In the short term we may see human embryonic tissue derived from excess embryos in IVF clinics, but if the political debate becomes too toxic the researchers will turn to other ways to make stem cell tissue.

For example, a researcher at the University of Massachusetts made an embryo-like thing by merging DNA from his cheek cells with a cow egg. He found what looked like stem cells in the resulting organism. Is that an embryo? Is it a chimera? Is it a clone? Is it human?

Second, what is the best way to regulate ethically difficult research? The answer clearly is not to play ostrich. Take infertility: Totally unregulated, research in infertility sometimes does not even require animal studies, and there are few rules about any of the important questions in the field.

Even with federal funding restored for stem cell research (after a hiatus during the Bush presidency), many argue that stem cell research still is hampered by existing federal regulations. With federal funding, the field is being controlled and the results carefully monitored. But some argue too carefully. This is why a significant portion of stem cell research in the United States is funded by the states – mainly California, New York, and Massachusetts.

Third, what is the right balance between respect for embryos and respect for the suffering patient? Sick Americans wait for the outcome of a debate about whether suffering ill, our parents and children, should be denied therapy when all that is required is that embryonic tissue is used in research rather than thrown away. This debate began in the late 1990s and continues to this day.

There isn't a debate here, there is the beginning of a critical conversation about the most important new technology of the millennium.

Everybody Lies

Case 9   Lies, Damn Lies . . . and Scientific Misconduct

Merriam Webster reported that in 2005, "integrity" received more hits than any other word in their online dictionary. This is highly ironic since it's not clear how many more hits scientific integrity can take: A MIT researcher is fired for fabricating a dozen papers. A pharmaceutical company omits data from key publications about side effects. A South Korean stem cell researcher admits to a stunned nation that "blinded by work and a drive for achievement," he submitted a "fake it before you make it" article to *Science*. It appears that research misconduct has taken its place among the epidemics that scientists need to worry about.

An aphorism attributed to Mark Twain holds that there are three kinds of lies: lies, damn lies, and statistics. At first the public points to a bad apple who paints mice or switches out slides and fumes if the researcher conspires to hide it. But it takes a village to do big science: authors, collaborators, students, sponsors, regulators; different languages, different countries, disparate goals. A lone scientist can offer mea culpa, but fraud on the scale of South Korea's almost always involves collusion and conspiracy, hidden in the complexity of the research. It is a nightmare for scientific journals, but more than anything it terrifies the public.

Science depends on public support. Too often, Hollywood sends the message to a fickle public that scientists-cum-fundraisers cannot be trusted to make what Malcolm Gladwell calls "blink" judgments about recruitment of egg donors, or to review thousands of pages of data. In the wake of the Hwang scandal in Korea, stem cell researchers who had been

Bioethics for Beginners: 60 Cases and Cautions from the Moral Frontier of Healthcare, First Edition. Glenn McGee.
© 2012 John Wiley & Sons, Ltd. Published 2012 by John Wiley & Sons, Ltd.

worshipped as heroes scraping for support become "rogues blinded by ambition." Those waging jihad against stem cell research talk about tangled webs, and they ask how far it is from an exaggeration of the results to an exaggeration of the benefits of embryonic cell research.

The solution to what the public – incorrectly – perceives as an epidemic of scientific misconduct is not obvious. Public relations is not the answer. Scientists who have spoken publicly about the Hwang matter have only made things worse. There are dozens of commissions on research ethics and programs to provide certification in it. There are conferences, journals, and agencies. Companies post ethics codes in hallways. Government pressure for compliance depends on funding, and in the United States, there's scant funding for stem cell research.

The great hope lies in teaching new generations of scientists, yet there's no evidence that it has an effect on the rate of misconduct. Scare tactics about the fate of Woo-suk Hwang will not transform those who enter graduate school ready to fabricate results, particularly when students report that their mentors could care less about the ethics course.

Nothing will prevent Dr. Jekyll from becoming Mr. Hyde, but mentors and oversight can help vulnerable newbies to science eschew bad habits. Researchers learn what is important by watching the boss; perhaps the boss should learn to teach the integrity course using lessons from the lab. Funding and institutional review-board approval should depend less on consent forms and more on ethics training and strategy. University compliance should emphasize remediation for those who play with matches rather than punishment for burning down the house.

Ultimately we don't have any clue what works, but it's a safe guess that the institutions that innovate in research ethics and study outcomes will be the ones that prevent misconduct. If we're going to throw buckets of money at frontier science, we'd better throw a little bit more at finding the best ways to help new scientists do it responsibly.

Case 10   Conflict of Interest Means Business at NIH

"NIH Announces Sweeping Ethics Reform," read a 2005 press release from Bethesda. The *Los Angeles Times* reported that "all staff scientists at the National Institutes of Health will be banned from accepting any consulting fees or other income from drug companies, and the employees must also divest industry stockholdings."

The old requirements, which put the greatest emphasis on self-reporting and made some awfully charitable assumptions when it comes to enforcement, could never have kept researchers at NIH clear of major conflicts of interest. It reminds me of the very poignant claim by Beecher all those years ago that the only way to really fix issues in research ethics is to teach researchers in a vastly less technocratic way than was (and is) the norm.

The focus is still on spankings for bad actions, rather than prophylactic ethics. Plus it relies upon a notion of culture shift that seems an anthema to scientific research. At a minimum, it means seriously going against the status quo where scientists were also employed by drug companies who benefited from their recommendations. Scientists endorsed treatments and new research at public meetings on the dime of the companies whose products they were endorsing.

The notion that all NIH scientists will be prohibited from accepting consulting fees, speaking fees, or any other form of income from any outside entity was pretty draconian indeed. Requiring scientists (and their spouses) to sell or otherwise dispose of any stock or stock options they hold in individual pharmaceutical or biotechnology firms just added insult to injury.

There is no NIH reputation problem bad enough to make me sell my stock

NIH employees quickly became furious over these "drastic" restrictions on stock ownership and other forms of outside income. Dr. Zerhouni met the critics of his new policy, saying "What I'm asking you to do is hold your fire until you hear the details."

They held. And when he was done, they let him have it.

One after another, scientists, doctors, and other agency staffers stepped up to the microphones and raged against the new rules. By the time it was over, 90 minutes later, nary a positive word had been uttered about the new policy and there was more vented spleen around than a busy medical center like the NIH might normally see in a year.

Clearly, Zerhouni made his best case. And he had one thing going for him: he is clearly right when he argues that aggressive rules on conflict of interest may be the key to "save the venerable agency's reputation, which had become badly sullied after 14 months of embarrassing revelations about conflicts of interest among NIH scientists."

But the policy asked for unmitigated selflessness on the part of every single NIH employee at the expense of people's college savings and nest eggs. And not all of these people in the NIH are susceptible to conflict of interest in the first place. Like the secretary of Ezekiel Emanuel, head of the NIH's bioethics department.

"Even my secretary is going to have to sell her stock. How much sense does that make?" fumed Emanuel.

But seriously, does Emanuel's secretary own more than $15,000 in drug, biotech and medical stocks? Because if she does, maybe she is conflicted given that she works for the ethics department at the NIH. Don't you wonder just a little bit how anybody can own more than $15,000 in pharma and biotech and medical stocks and be utterly immune to the power that being in the world's brain center for medicine brings?

But there were other concerns from scientists at NIH that flat out make sense. One NIH section chief put it bluntly, "Does this apply to the Department of Energy? To the Department of Agriculture? To the Defense Department?" Her question was met with cheers and applause.

"If we really want to reassure the public," Emanuel added, "why don't we apply these to everyone who gets an NIH grant?"

Again applause.

Another attendee noted that NIH employees are subject to periodic outside evaluations and reviews by nongovernmental scientists who are not subject to the same ethics restrictions – a bizarre situation, the employee said, in which people with real conflicts of interest will be sitting in judgment of those with none.

Moreover, the NIH calls upon hundreds of outside scientists from academia and industry to judge grant proposals every year – people who have far more power over purse strings than most employees but who will not be covered by the new rules.

That speaker was among several who refused to identify themselves to reporters because of fears of punishment by superiors at the Department of Health and Human Services. One told a reporter that employees were being "muzzled." Another said "there have been retributions." Neither would elaborate.

Still others complained that the stock restrictions will apply not only to themselves but to their spouses, as well. "Spouses are independent people," one researcher explained. He added that his wife has already contacted the American Civil Liberties Union to discuss the issue.

Clearly, attempting to resolve conflicts of interest has created much more conflict than anyone would have anticipated. And the most important question, left unanswered, is whether this new policy will accomplish its stated goal of removing financial bias among researchers at the NIH. That still remains to be seen.

Case 11 While You're Here, How about a Spinal Tap?

Evidence has mounted that Duke and other major medical research universities do not take enough care in protecting research subjects. At Duke, inspectors found that research subjects were never followed up to see what was happening, and that the institution's research ethics review board did not follow up on studies that it approved. Was it carelessness or something else?

With tremendous cuts in Medicaid, the pressure is on big universities to do more and more human research that can make up the money lost in federal subsidies. Unless the research oversight capacity expands at the same rate as the addition of new human subjects research, it can be no surprise that things will fall through the cracks.

A *New York Times* investigative report found the same problem in little clinics around the nation: physicians, with earnings decreasing, are turning to pharmaceutical research to supplement their income. Around the nation, individual physicians are jumping on the band-wagon of research as well, taking big bucks from "clinical research organizations" to sign up their sick and healthy patients for studies, sometimes misleading their patients to boost enrollment. Many physicians take cash or other rewards to enroll patients in studies that may or may not benefit the patient. It is increasingly clear that patients and research subjects don't have much clue how much money is exchanged, or about the precautions that are being taken on their behalf by physicians, health maintenance organizations (HMOs), universities, and the government.

It is a big problem. There aren't anywhere near enough subjects to test the barrage of new drugs and devices that have come out of the recent boom in American pharmacology research.

Most Americans are very proud of US leadership in pharmaceuticals, but not many volunteer to help test the research unless there is some personal incentive. Patients typically volunteer to enroll in studies of potential drugs that they (or their physicians) believe could help them.

21

If I am depressed but can't afford psychotherapy, I might enroll in a free study of a potential antidepressant. If all my efforts to fight a cancer have failed, I may search the world and empty my bank accounts in an effort to enroll in a study of a potential anti-cancer agent.

Healthy Americans volunteer when they see signs in newspapers and subways and hear ads on the radio offering cash for participation. But there still aren't enough volunteers. So medical research has become, largely, a business.

New rules

The rules of the new research game are much more complicated than they used to be. Before World War II, most research subjects were patients, and we rarely made a distinction between those two roles. Today, law and ethical rules attempt to make a distinction between the roles of physician and researcher, and the roles of patient and subject.

Before 1980, researchers who were funded by federal money had a hard time partnering with companies, and most clinical research was conducted in universities. After the passage of the Bayh–Dole Act of 1980, many universities began partnering up with big companies and the government. It is almost impossible to tell where the public money stops and big business begins.

For most of the twentieth century, the population that was exposed to clinical research trials was pretty much limited to the sick and those otherwise vulnerable: children, the institutionalized and members of minority groups. Today just about anyone with time to kill and empty pockets is a potential research subject, with the result that lots of people – and more to come – are taking on a second job as guinea pig.

The problem of course is that US research institutions don't protect research subjects very well. Confronted with a 10-page "informed consent" form and a high-pressure sales pitch, vulnerable Americans enroll every day in studies that expose them to real danger without sufficient safeguards.

It is time for a national overhaul of our clinical research system, and time to put ethics first.

Case 12   Study Subject or Human Guinea Pig?

Every day more than a million Americans put in a day's work as foot soldiers in the drive to discover. They are research subjects, and they volunteer their services for many reasons. Many are ill and join to try a new approach to their disease.

Many are poor and join a research program to earn extra money. Some are unable to get health insurance and turn to researchers to get a little bit of mental healthcare or prenatal care as part of a study. Some are children, some are aging, some are from faraway indigenous populations.

The buzzword for protecting these subjects of research is "informed consent." Presidential commissions, Nazi trials and the United Nations all have endorsed the uniform requirement that competent adult research subjects be informed about all aspects of the risks of the research and given uncoerced consent to participate.

"Tough, ambiguous job"

In the United States, universities and corporations alike use institutional review boards (IRBs) to review proposals for research involving human subjects. Their job is to protect everyone involved, from subjects to their families to the institutions who sponsor research. The IRB must figure out whether research is safe, is ready to go to human trials and is being described accurately to potential subjects. It is a tough, ambiguous job and the only requirement for membership in an IRB is that you say "yes" to joining.

As successful as research has become in our century, just about everyone agrees there are problems with the way we treat human subjects. In the *Journal of the American Medical Association*, a team of ethicists and clinicians in a special task force on research ethics at the University of Pennsylvania in Philadelphia proposed some dramatic changes to the way we regulate research.

It is about time.

Among the panel's conclusions: Informed consent documents, long and cumbersome, should be replaced by a careful and interactive process. IRBs should be part of a much more careful system designed to prevent the use of guinea pigs who have not been adequately informed or who have coerced by desperation, lack of adequate medical insurance or unrealistic hopes for a cure. It is time to lead the way in the world of protecting human test subjects.

Case 13   The New Tuskegee: Exploiting the Poor in Clinical Trials

In one among a series of exposés (they appear somewhere every year or so) of the clinical trials industry, Bloomberg news service reveals (yet again) something that drives me crazy. Quoting astonished ethicists – including Ken Goodman of the University of Miami, whom the reporter brought to a clinical trials site – the reporters identify one of many clinical trials sites engaged in truly ugly exploitation of research subjects.

The setting is laid out like a script for a play (and indeed several plays have focused on clinical research abuses):

> Oscar Cabanerio has been waiting in an experimental drug testing center in Miami since 7:30 a.m. The 41-year-old undocumented immigrant says he is desperate for cash to send his wife and four children in Venezuela.
>
> More than 70 people have crowded into reception rooms furnished with rows of attached blue plastic seats. Cabanerio is one of many regulars who gather at SFBC International Inc.'s test center, which, with 675 beds, is the largest for-profit drug testing center in North America. Most of the people lining up at SFBC to rent their bodies to medical researchers are poor immigrants from Latin America, drawn to this five-story test center in a converted Holiday Inn motel.
>
> Inside, the brown paint and linoleum is gouged and scuffed. A bathroom with chipped white tiles reeks of urine; its floor is covered with muddy footprints and used paper towels. The volunteers, who are supposed to be healthy, wait for the chance to get paid for ingesting chemicals that might make them sick.
>
> They are testing the compounds that the world's largest pharmaceutical companies hope to develop into best-selling medicines. Cabanerio, who has a mechanical drafting degree from a technical school, says he left Venezuela because he lost his job as a union administrator. For him, the visit to SFBC is a last resort. "I'm in a bind," Cabanerio said in Spanish. "I need the money."

The poor, who are most vulnerable are being offered cash and promises of therapeutic efficacy ("depressed? got no money for psychotherapy? we will give you free evaluations and study medications ...") to serve as faceless guinea pigs in multiple and poorly policed experiments in labs that boggle the mind. Troy Duster famously referred to "credit card eugenics," a new form of genetic selection dominated by a market rather than the state. I submit that clinical trials in the United States have become a "welfare Tuskegee."

Not only African Americans, and not only a small town, and not with the deliberate and systematic involvement of public health authorities, there is nonetheless a broad and even systematic campaign that is ongoing to design clinical trials – the ads, the facilities, the trials themselves and the cash payments – in such away as to deceive and endanger specific and well understood socioeconomic groups in society.

The regulations are "porous" enough so that some medical centers have had non-physicians conduct clinical trials for years with bogus credentials – faking a medical degree for example. The solutions proposed in bioethics to date have been less than imaginative, and nobody is stepping up to the plate from policy or pharma either.

In fact the single most apparent change in clinical trials has been the divestment of pharma in the clinical trials industry: one large pharmaceutical company after another has decided that the best idea is to outsource them for lower cost – and to eliminate liability.

It is a new version of an old problem and we need to go from being astonished to being furious. Even if that means fighting your own university's psychiatry department, or developing new roles that feel more like "ethics police" than like researchers. And I am skeptical enough to suspect that it is fear of our own institutions – most of whom benefit mightily from clinical trials – that plays a big role in preventing many of us in bioethics from studying or protesting research ethics abuses in our own institutions. The most prominent case of resisting that kind of pressure was that of Mary Faith Marshall (now of University of Minnesota), who famously fought against State sanctioned abuse of pregnant women in South Carolina and paid a significant penalty as a result.

Bioethics has been asleep at this switch for too long, teaching responsible research courses that hang on the Tuskegee experiment as though we have come so far in fifty years. Come so far? Tell that to Oscar Cabanerio. India, one of the worst offenders in research ethics for years, has done more to reform clinical trials than the United States.

Something must be done to stop this exploitation. I cannot believe I am saying this, given my skepticism about national commissions in bioethics and their utter lack of effectiveness in recent years, but it is time for a national commission on clinical trials that focuses on these issues. Or better yet it would be great if a senator took up the challenge, as happened (to terrible effect, granted) in 1993 concerning emergency research. The commission should be – minimally sponsored by the Institute of Medicine and the American Society of Bioethics and Humanities. Perhaps then we would, at least, surpass developing world countries in regard to the protections we provide to research subjects.

25

Case 14 Salt in the Wound: Will India Rise up Against the Oppression of Foreign Clinical Trials?

In March 1930, Mohandas Gandhi set out from his ashram in western India on a 387-km trek to the sea. Twenty-five days later the tens of thousands who joined that march watched as he stooped, raised a handful of salty mud, and declared the end of British imperialism in India. The march culminated as Gandhi led nonviolent protesters to the doors of the salt factory in Dharasana, where they attempted to push their way into the facility without weapons or raised fists. On that hot day hundreds were beaten, a spectacle that would make its way into newspapers worldwide and change the face of India forever.

If Gandhi were alive today, I am confident that he would lead protesters to the doors of Indian clinical research trials facilities. Why? Not because Gandhi was a Luddite, a man who held meetings while spinning thread. And not because many of the excellent research institutions that have led India into its embrace of multinational bioengineering and medical research bear his family name.

No, the problem for Gandhi would be the outsourced clinical trials that have enrolled tens of thousands of Indians in a $1 billion business aimed not at the improvement of Indians' health or technology, but at providing deep discounts to pharmaceutical companies in other nations. It would be the oppression of the Indian poor which dwarfs that of the 1930s for the benefit of research imperialists.

It is a perfect storm: The number of open slots in clinical trials around the world increases, the number of Americans willing to enroll in such trials lags (as few as 1.7 percent of patients with cancer), and the cost of clinical trials in India is half that in the United States. It is no surprise that American and European pharmaceutical companies are fanning out across the second most populous nation in the world.

Physicians in India report that a largely illiterate subject population, entirely unclear about risks and benefits, asks only one question: Doctor, should I enroll? At least one study in the *Indian Journal of Medical Ethics* reported that many Indian research subjects are utterly unprepared to distinguish between trials likely to provide benefit and those that will not.

According to a 2005 report in the *New England Journal of Medicine*, fewer than 200 of the 14,000 general hospitals in India are capable of conducting clinical trials adequately.

Why do Indians, most of whom are poor, flock to clinical trials? One reason is that most of the nation is served by small and ill-equipped hospitals where they fail to get adequate or any treatment. The "chambers of commerce" for clinical trials in India point to the advantages of this fact: Indian patients are often untreated, reducing the number of confounding factors in study of medications. And a tiny payment, by US standards, to an Indian enrollee in a clinical trial could amount to three months' wages or more. Incentive payments to physicians for enrolling research subjects are also amplified greatly by the exchange rate. Plus, clinical trials provide Indians with access to the medical care that they desperately need. A win-win, right?

Wrong.

The government attempted in 2004 to rein in unsafe international clinical trials by insisting that drugs tested in India must first be proven safe in their country of origin. But that law was eliminated in 2005, followed closely by an avalanche of new trials. Concerns about trials that are designed to demonstrate nominally important data, are poorly designed, or are just plain unsafe abound. Some trials are conducted on humans without prior animal studies having been performed. In one unapproved clinical trial for example, 435 women were given an anticancer drug to treat fertility, but did not know the drug was not cleared for this use.

The same imperialism that supported the salt factories of Dharasana in 1930 today manifests itself in Mumbai, Sevagram, and around India, where clinical trials too offensive for American research subjects are proffered to a billion residents of the nation Gandhi fought so hard to emancipate. How long before the people in the nation of Gandhi rise up to reject this new imperialism?

Case 15   Dr. Hwang and the Bad Apple
Theory of Scientific Misconduct

The lone liar theory

Several of my favorite colleagues, including Laurie Zoloth in the *Los Angeles Times*, have distilled the ethical implications of the Hwang matter to "telling the truth."

Laurie writes:

The bottom line is this: In a complicated world, the public must trust experts, because how can you know what to do if you cannot know what is real? Tell the truth, always, we teach students, withhold nothing from your data. It is a categorical imperative for science and indeed for all societies. It comes from Immanuel Kant, whose early writings on truth in the new discipline of science shaped what we teach as core questions in bioethics . . . Bioethicists cannot reflect on complex moral issues without a truthful narrative. Policymakers cannot regulate without good facts. The public cannot know what to hope for if it cannot know what is real.

The submission of an article for publication in a science journal may well be, as David Magnus points out, a form of testimony. But whose testimony is it? Who must stand to account for the science that seems to have been literally made up in this paper? In this case more than 20 authors. And several institutions. And high-ranking government officials.

To be sure, if the allegations are demonstrated in South Korea, the alleged activities in this case would join Summerlin's painted mice and the Piltdown "missing link" man in the Great Halls of Bogus Discovery. But there is an important difference in this case. In this case a legion of collaborators share the responsibility. The lone-liar theory falls apart. As was reported in a December 2005 article in the *Korea Times*:

> the Board of Audit and Investigation has requested the Ministry of Science and Technology submit documents on the state funding it has provided to Hwang's research team . . . The state auditor's probe into the ministry is expected to focus on the ministry's management of Hwang's research fund and the government's report channels on the destruction of several stem cells that Hwang reported in January.

In addition, its probe is targeting the Ministry of Health and Welfare for its subsides worth $15 billion won provided for construction of the World Stem Cell Hub . . . The inspection agency is also looking into $4.3 billion won in subsidies offered in 2001 to Wang's research team by the Ministry of Information and Communication.

This case will turn out to be like peeling an onion.

Hwang's lab was subject to extreme funding mechanisms, insufficient oversight, excessive pressure, a crazy confederation of authors and institutions, confusion about patents, translation of both language and data by international collaborators, pressures from peers (the so-called "chopstick theory of scientific supremacy") and more importantly from the culture, and a grossly irresponsible lack of American leadership in the regulatory and funding arena where in virtue of our intellectual property, our consumer safety rules, and our national interest in getting the science right we have that responsibility.

We in bioethics are part of the problem. We undertake partnership with and are often seen as giving approval to the companies, agencies, industry organizations and individuals that share our ideals, and sometimes the enemy of our enemy is our friend. This is true whether we heading their ethics committees, as I once did for an American stem cell company, or working in their industry organizations. In my own case the company whom I was helping failed to inform me that it was doing cloning experiments that were of profound moral significance ... a fact I found out when I was asked to comment on the experiments for a news organization. In this case Laurie details with equal regret standing alongside Hwang for an announcement where validation of the significance and ethics of the experiment mattered a great deal. And John Robertson wrote persuasively in this blog, in commenting on what he saw as hyperventilation about the egg donation problem in Hwang's lab, that, "Now that [Hwang] has done his public mea culpa I say the time is to forgive him and let him get back to plying his considerable craft."

No. Lying is bad. But the tangled web in this matter is not the sort of thing one finds in the history of scientific misconduct. An entirely new kind of deception occurred here, one in which picking out the key player will be like playing "Where's Waldo."

The implosion of Korean stem cell research

Gerald P. Schatten, who has taken the lead in American collaboration with Korea's leader in stem cell research, pulled out of that collaboration because of what he referred to as ethical breaches and lies.

Schatten's allegation – which became a huge scandal in Korea – involves the way that Hwang and his colleagues obtained the eggs that they used in making the embryos from which they harvested stem cells. According to Rick Weiss at the *Washington Post*:

> For many months after Hwang's 2004 publication, rumors had spread in scientific circles that the eggs Hwang used to achieve that landmark result had been taken from a junior scientist in his lab. That situation, if true, would be in violation of widely held ethics principles that preclude people in positions of authority from accepting egg donations from underlings. The rules are meant to prevent subtle – or not-so-subtle – acts of coercion. Questions have also circulated as to whether the woman received illegal payments for her role. Schatten said that Hwang had repeatedly denied the

rumor and that he had believed Hwang until yesterday. "I now have information that leads me to believe he had misled me," Schatten said. "My trust has been shaken. I am sick at heart. I am not going to be able to collaborate with Woo Suk."

So what, you might say, if one Korean researcher makes a mistake and it leads to the discontinuation of one partnership between a group in Seoul and a guy from Pittsburgh. Well it is much bigger than that. The impact of the continuing catastrophe with the Hwang lab is not, of course, because he used cloning to create Snuppy the dog.

Hwang's work has been revolutionary in the scientific quest to do "therapeutic cloning" – to use nuclear transfer in order to make embryonic stem cell lines, and to do it more efficiently and faster than anyone thought possible. He has made them in strange ways, to be sure, such as deriving the somatic cells from six-year olds.

And Hwang is a symbol – big time. The unmitigated praise for his "Korean work ethic" many have cited as the reason for his incredible success. He alone had made progress with the Catholic Church on how to proceed with stem cell research. Anyone who was paying attention to that moment would have noted the stark contrast between Hwang's careful approach and that of those in the United States who have instead decided to play semantic games or do bizarre science in order to avoid the debate.

He alone received more money from the Korean government than the US government has given out everyone put together for research using the President's approved stem cell lines.

But most – including Schatten – believed that the bulk of his research involved derivation of stem cell lines from materials that had been properly donated under careful scrutiny. What do I mean by "most"? Well, to put it in a nutshell, Woo Suk's effort has just last month culminated in the announcement that his team plans to create hundreds of stem cell lines every year. Many of us in bioethics, though, quietly took notice that while the Schatten group – who had been working with Hwang for a while – linked up early and consistently with Hwang, other major stem cell researchers were cautious. And when the big explosion happened in Korea, it became clear that the Pitt agreement with Hwang was doomed.

I would have said – and in fact most major news and technology magazines have written – that Hwang's team has become the one to beat in the "stem cell race," and that his efforts to think about ethics of stem cell research were unmatched even among the California scientists who must now create and follow highly complex regulations about egg donation.

But Hwang's misleading Schatten, the Korean government, the Catholic Church – who really went the distance in listening to and trusting him, and the people in his lab, was tragic in a way that vastly exceeds the simple violations of research ethics.

Hwang firmly established in the public mind the view that stem cell researchers as a group cannot be trusted, not only because they are in a hurry and miss things along the way, but because they may be willing to deceive their own peers and the public about their devotion to ethics. Stem cell researchers do good work, and many of them are very thoughtful about the controversy that attends it. But the bar is higher. Embryonic stem cell research, research that involves the donation of eggs, and particularly research that involves therapeutic cloning simply demands that scientists show the utmost respect to everyone involved and the utmost trustworthiness about how they proceed.

If this doesn't prove that there needed to be a program to study legal and social issues in stem cell research, I cannot imagine what would. And in the meantime, it is going to be a rough few ... well, forevers, for Korean stem cell research. And it remains an open question whether Hwang can stay out of jail or not.

Because there is no real federal funding for embryonic stem cell research, other nations have begun to take the lead. But the real concern isn't that the other guys are winning, it is what happens when they bend the rules to do so.

Hwang Woo-suk is South Korea's first superstar scientist. His team was the first to successfully make stem cells using cloned human embryos – a process often referred to as therapeutic cloning. He has been busy since his initial breakthrough.

Since creating the first cloned human embryos, he created a technique to derive stem cells five times more efficiently using far fewer donated eggs. Last April he held a news conference at which a stem cell research subject walked after having been bedridden for 19 years. Hwang is also the scientific father to the world's second-most-famous cloned animal, Snuppy the dog.

South Korea took notice of his work. The grateful Asian nation of 48 million has lavished praise, titles, and money on Hwang, declaring him their first "supreme scientist." His labs receive more support than the US government has invested in all of our nation's stem cell labs put together.

It should be no surprise then that a leading American stem cell scientist, Gerald Schatten, wanted to work with Hwang. Finding a partner overseas was a matter of survival for Schatten's University of Pittsburgh team, because embryonic stem cell research is a third-degree felony in Pennsylvania.

An impressive work ethic prevails in South Korea. Hwang's labs do not close – ever. He has said that all of his scientists work every day of the week. Their devotion and his success, he jokes, derives from the "chopstick theory of scientific supremacy," by which he means that because Korean chopsticks are metal and somewhat slippery, one has to learn early to be precise. While Dr. Hwang's work ethics may be impressive, his research ethics may be less so.

One key requirement for success in therapeutic cloning to create stem cells is raw material. Cloners need eggs. To make Snuppy the dog, Korean scientists used more than 1,000 dog eggs to create embryos which they transferred into 123 dogs to create one Snuppy.

Hwang and Schatten's work in making human embryonic cells required an unprecedented amount of human eggs. Since the odds against any single cloned embryo working are enormous, they needed a lot of eggs to make a lot of embryos.

That means that many women would need to be willing to consent to the risks of taking hormones so they would create a lot of eggs and then having them removed surgically from their ovaries. And that is where things went wrong.

Schatten announced recently that he would no longer be collaborating with Hwang. He cited new information that led him to believe that Hwang's group had accepted eggs from a young woman who is a junior scientist in the lab. He also said he had evidence that the woman may have been paid for her eggs.

Taking eggs from an employee smacks of coercion. Paying for them smacks of bad judgment. If Hwang's lab knowingly violated the rights of egg donors in a rush to advance stem cell research, and then when asked about such behavior, covered it up, a lot of people will start asking whether or not stem cell researchers are a rogue lot, not to be trusted. What is the answer? Get the US government involved in paying for and regulating embryonic stem cell research.

A clear majority of Americans favor embryonic stem cell research. Yet there are no meaningful federal funds for such research. And the administration has been growling about cloning for research ever since it took office.

As a result, our best stem cell researchers, like Professor Schatten, going offshore to avoid prosecution or to find research funds.

This means that ethics can get forgotten as other nations and private companies race to fill the void left by the president's reluctance to fund stem cell research.

Only a properly funded US stem cell research program will guarantee oversight and the protection of all involved. Professor Hwang has gotten too powerful and the Korean government too dazzled with his work to allow him to be a sole man in Seoul.

Caution **Three**

The Genome Isn't What It Used to Be

Case 16   Becoming Genomic: Just What Does it Mean Anyway?

The ticker tape parades and high-wattage celebrations of the mapping of the human genome are being replaced, if you listen to those who gather around the coffee pot in America's top scientific labs, by discussions of epigenetic research, the microbiome, and synthetic biology. But even if the scientists have moved on, the rest of us are just beginning to understand how fast and how far genetic research has come. The world of genomics represents the most significant shift in our lifestyle since the adoption of personal computers.

If you are like me, you won't be able to read the articles about the human genome in the prestigious journals *Nature* and *Science*. To those untrained in genetics, the articles are no more comprehensible than the actual DNA code itself – TAC, CTA, GAS and so on – the various three-letter combinations, strung together in various forms, carrying the instructions for making all organisms. Maybe that's an overly simplified explanation, but you get it: The fact that we can't read them is the point.

The trick to understanding genomics is that long strings of genetic information are becoming linked to one another and to complex information about human health. Not all of this information is about the genes that you inherit – genomics also deals with the effect that viruses, mutagens, and aging have on genes, and the effect that damaged genomes have on organisms.

Bioethics for Beginners: 60 Cases and Cautions from the Moral Frontier of Healthcare,
First Edition. Glenn McGee.
© 2012 John Wiley & Sons, Ltd. Published 2012 by John Wiley & Sons, Ltd.

Genomics has introduced new concepts about genetics, but more importantly it has taken most of the work of genetics out of the lab and replaced it with something that looks a lot more like computer programming than "bench" science.

In giant "computer farms," software and hardware turn bits of human cells into massive databases, and the resulting genomic programs are rapidly working their way into every aspect of human life.

Genetics was an interesting but complex science that explained how we inherit particular traits. Genomics is a shift in how we see ourselves, our potential, our families and our society.

It is also a business, a much faster moving kind of science that has vastly outstripped our social conversation about genetics.

Like the evolution of live music first into albums, then into CDs and now onto the Internet, the development of genomics is happening very quickly. Ten years ago it would have been unthinkable for a healthy woman to remove her own breasts because her mother had breast cancer. Today a genomic aberration is often the most real thing about a disease, and it can be patented (perhaps), emailed and traded on the stock market.

The transition to being genomic is part of a transition to a more digital lifestyle. My genes will soon fit on the digital chip implanted in a smart card in my wallet, so clinicians can easily refer to it when I get sick.

Prevention-based medicine

Already the first sign of genomic living is in full bloom: Society has moved from medicine based on disease to medicine based on susceptibility and prevention. Eventually, for less than $1,000, a doctor will swab a few cells from inside your cheek, pop them into a DNA sequencing machine and, voila, a computer will spit out a complete reading of your unique genetic makeup – all 30,000 of your genes, together called your genome. From that, physicians can pinpoint flawed genes, predicting what diseases you are likely to develop years in advance of any symptoms and prescribing drug therapy based on your genetic makeup.

Drugs are already being tested to identify whose genome is best for what agent. Is your genome antidepressant-resistant? Does your wife's genome mean she cannot eat steak, or your neighbor's mean that he is more likely to spread deadly infections? Understanding how your genome puts you at extra risk or special advantage will be a critical part of being genomic.

On its way are answers to new kinds of questions: about genomic privacy, about the ownership of our genomes and about what kind of babies will be born in the genomic era. Will parents take advantage of genomics to improve upon their children's traits?

As genomics continues to develop in the next decade, its influence on agriculture, computing, manufacturing, education and politics will expand even more.

So what should we as a society be doing?

New laws about genetic privacy and discrimination are a good start, but without a way to understand the new operating system of genomics, we are a lot like the astronaut Dave confronting the famous computer HAL in Stanley Kubrick's classic movie about technology out of control, a film aptly named *2001*.

We don't really know how to turn genomics on or off, and we can't quite figure out whether it is working for us or against us. Only one thing is certain about the New World of genomics: The time has come to begin talking about what it means to be genomic.

Case 17 Enhancement Comes from Insecurity

University of Minnesota's Carl Elliott wins the "best title" award hands down for "This Is Your Country on Drugs" in the *New York Times*.[1] The platform is steroids, but his article is about the evils of enhancement technology more generally. He writes:

> Jacques Barzun famously said that to understand America, one must first understand baseball. Never has his remark been more accurate. Professional baseball players may be the most vilified Americans using performance-enhancing drugs, but they are by no means alone. Performance-enhancing drugs have become a part of ordinary American life.

Sounds interesting, right? But this prominent op-ed about the dangers of enhancement is full of fear and trembling, in the key of "repugnance," toting the line that enhancement is self-denial. Elliott uses the clever anti-enhancement language he has popularized, and that is now trumpeted by Leon Kass, former chair of President Bush Jr.'s President's Council on Bioethics and fellow at the American Enterprise Institute, (e.g., to attempt to deal with a faltering memory is to try to be "better than well"), and commits all Kass' fallacies, most importantly failing to define what "well" means.

The upshot of Elliott's argument is thus pretty puritanical, substituting Luddite condemnation of an enhancement "industry" for an appraisal of changing ideas about the meaning of disease. It is easy to describe steroid use by baseball players as non-medical, and clearly the physicians who prescribe those medications using libido as a diagnosis are not acting responsibly. But steroids for baseball players are a far cry from Viagra for help with sex. Elliott does not bother to argue for the incredibly implausible link he draws from such behavior to performance enhancements that more properly fit within a medical sphere. So it is no surprise that he is able to conclude that enhancement is a pitiful band aid for the soul: "America's appetite for stimulants, antidepressants and Botox injections looks less like enthusiasm and more like fear." But the connection between baseball and makeup doesn't really lead where Carl thinks it does.

People improve themselves all the time, and there is no more human struggle than that to improve one's own, and others', quality of life. That struggle defines much of parenthood, for example, as I argued in a book called *The Perfect Baby*.

You have to ignore a lot of human experience to demonize all enhancement technologies as a "desire to avoid shame and humiliation," rather than a desire to succeed. Exercise is based on a desire to succeed but a facelift is based on shame? Not always. Plenty of people exercise out of shame, to the point even that they reduce their lives to a thin gruel. Many people take showers, put on powder, and buy clothes because they want to look "better," but not because they are ashamed and miserable and humiliated.

When you shake out Elliott's (and Kass') arguments about enhancement, they boil down to repugnance, not as much at technology as at habits that offend Kass' and Elliott's sensibilities. This will come as no surprise to those who have read Kass' incredibly conservative writing about food and sex. The danger is that this kind of argument will be viewed as nothing more than patronizing claptrap by most of those who want to use enhancement technology, and thus does nothing whatever to help institutions and individuals put enhancement in context. Abject loathing of any "weird new technologies" for the desire to improve ourselves actually hurts the effort to discern between enhancements that should be slowed, or banned, and those that make a lot of sense.

Case 18 Wearing Genes from the Gulf War

Some veterans of the Gulf War have ribonucleic acid (RNA), which the body employs to make proteins, in the serum that carries their blood cells, reported Urnovitz's team at the Chronic Illness Research Foundation and California-based Calypte Biomedical Corporation.

It had been thought that RNA could not survive outside a cell or virus. Urnovitz hypothesized that pesticides, oil smoke, chemical warfare agents and other toxins may have caused some veterans' immune systems to rearrange the DNA in some of our cells, so-called memory cells.

Memory cells are a tool of the immune system, enabling our bodies to recognize familiar invaders (say, a virus you inhaled on a commercial airplane) and then respond quickly. Unusual memory cells may have been created by exposure to toxic chemicals in the Gulf. These cells, Urnovitz believes, created a strange RNA that acts like a virus and is able to survive in serum.

This RNA could cause cancer, birth defects in offspring, or autoimmune disorders, he says. None of this explains a single "Gulf War Disease." But the implications of genetic change like that observed by Urnovitz are mind-blowing.

Urnovitz and his team seem to be saying something baffling: Gulf War syndrome may be genetic. Many scientists and doctors and most Americans think of genetics as the "language of life," our destiny encoded in DNA. We are born with genes, right?

So is Urnovitz actually saying that Gulf War syndrome is inherited? Not exactly. Rather, Urnovitz's research points to the fact that genes aren't just something you are born with. The genes in your cells may come from your parents, but those same genes can be changed by the environments in which you live and work.

Much of the Gulf War syndrome may turn out to be genetic. But that doesn't mean veterans are born with the syndrome. We are learning that while many causes of disease are genetic, not all genetic problems are hereditary.

We know of more and more diseases that involve a genetic change, caused by something in the environment. Our genes can change. And you have to be careful where you wear them.

We are a long way from understanding what symptoms the Gulf War caused. But we are beginning to realize how important it is to study not only the genes we are born with, but also the genetic changes that happen to people as a result of the world in which they live.

Some genetic changes are really unpredictable, and no one sets out to cause a genetic change like the kind seen in cancer or the symptoms reported by some Gulf War veterans. But when lots of folks have the same genetic changes, it isn't just a mutation anymore.

It is a genetic disease caused by a dangerous environment.

The challenge of genetics in this millennium isn't just figuring out what your genes do. It is figuring out how to wear your genes: what causes them to change and what those changes mean.

Learning about changes in genes will be a tall order, but we owe it to the future generations, folks who will also wear genes.

Note

1. Elliott's article was published December 14, 2004.

Caution **Four**

Reproduce at Your Own Peril

Case 19   Tomorrow's Child: Making Babies in the Twenty-First Century

Prediction

The next century will welcome some pretty unusual bundles of joy. Your next child will come from the stork, but your great-grandchildren may be engineered in a computer lab. In years to come, we will see human clones, babies with cyborg implants and the combination of human and animal tissues for a variety of purposes. Progress will come at the cost of today's ideas about what a family means. Tomorrow's idea of family may look a lot more like a hive.

Babies of the future

There are lots of improvements we might wish for. Babies with sweet-smelling diapers who sleep all night will be in great demand. Children are incredibly vulnerable and what parent won't want a tiny, implanted monitoring system to keep track of vital statistics and growth? Today we "have" our babies, using a time honored method called "sex." But couples who today choose designer sperm donors, sex selection and big-bucks private school are paving the way for tomorrow's child: a baby whose DNA is made from "the best" available genes.

Remember the birds and the bees? History. Or rather, hobby. Tomorrow's couples will have lots of reasons to separate sex from making babies. Sex will always be, well, an enjoyable part of partnership. But tomorrow's "act of love" that relates to making babies may feel more like

Bioethics for Beginners: 60 Cases and Cautions from the Moral Frontier of Healthcare,
First Edition. Glenn McGee.
© 2012 John Wiley & Sons, Ltd. Published 2012 by John Wiley & Sons, Ltd.

negotiating over how to build a house: blonde or brunette? Tall or short? Poet's disposition or quarterback's metabolism? And you won't be the only one pushing for an improvement. It costs a lot of money to be tall. Short is much more efficient. And for that matter, wouldn't it be better if human beings could digest cellulose, so we could eat lower on the food chain?

Tomorrow's environmental movement may be as much about reducing the local consumption of the human body as about preserving the distant rain forest.

It is expensive to have hereditary predisposition to disease. It costs big bucks to have many children. Lots of our habits might be better served by a more resilient heart, lungs, and brain. And if you think your life is nothing but work today, imagine implanting telecommunications, data transfer, and enhanced entertainment directly into your brain. "Dad, can I install a PSNeuro? I promise to think about my homework most of the time!"

All of these things and many more I cannot imagine will go from science fiction to the laboratory before your great-grandchildren are born.

Politics of genetics

The politics of genetic modification is about fear, money, and religion. Fear is much more an issue for adults than kids. Today's kids are fascinated by the idea of cloning and look expectantly to a world they can help shape and improve.

What bioethicist Arthur Caplan calls the "yuck factor" is a phenomenon of fear at times of transition from one kind of world to another. Fear fades. Money motivates change in biomedicine and today you have only to look at the geography of any leading health center to see how much things are already moving ahead. See that new building at the University? It's pretty much guaranteed that it says "GENETICS" on the front door. We are investing in a future of genetic decision-making and it would be folly to think that none of this technology will reach parents.

Money also motivates employers and even employees when we pick our insurance and our medical care. If an insurance company decided to decline payment for a baby with a hereditary disease, the nation would go nuts. But in the next century medical institutions will certainly offer the reverse: discounts for families who take high-tech precautions that result in a less expensive birth.

41

Faith and morality

Let's start telling our children stories about the future to help them imagine a world that will be exciting but full of ethical challenges.

Finally, religion is changing, and changing fast. The politics of "Leave it to Beaver" family values, for twenty years dominated by right-wing religious action groups, simply will not hold up in a world where the new options are so attractive to people of many faiths. Moreover, the science of yesterday's battles is changing. The old debates about abortion, for example, make assumptions about how babies are made that just don't apply anymore. Cloned mammals aren't conceived, and most of them don't make it to birth. Are they embryos? The major religious groups just aren't sure yet.

I don't worry about designer babies forming armies and to takeover the world. I don't worry about dictators making clones to pilot secret planes. And I am not terrified late at night that my offspring will want to rid the world of imperfect people like me. What does scare me is the total lack of social dialogue about genetic improvement.

It is time for town hall meetings about genetics, reproduction, and the future of the family. It is time to train everyone from librarians to primary school teachers to clergy to think about these issues too. Most importantly, it is time to start telling our children stories about the future to help them imagine a world that will be exciting, but challenging too.

Case 20   An Argument against Human Cloning

It is patent that human cloning should not proceed to the clinical research stage. A moratorium on clinical trials of human cloning is warranted on safety grounds, as there is no pathway from animal to pre-clinical to clinical human experimentation that would not involve significant risks to human children. As we have noted elsewhere, it is doubtful even in the long term that an individual or couple will present a rationale for the use of human cloning technologies that is compelling when balanced against the risks.[1] Here we argue that social restrictions on human cloning can best be justified and implemented on the model of law and policy about adoption.

Regulation and debate about human reproduction may be modeled on three different emphases. We will call these models the reproductive freedom model, the pediatric model, and the adoption model.

This century has seen the birth of an entirely new kind of jurisprudence about sexuality and reproduction. Fueled by scientific developments like birth control and in vitro fertilization, and against the backdrop of international civil rights reform, courts in the twentieth century framed a new dimension of the freedom of expression: the right to choose one's progeny. The right to make one's own decisions about reproduction has several strata. A right against government interference in reproduction is most clearly codified in American case law about discontinuation of pregnancy. *Roe vs. Wade* and *Casey* carve out a right to reproductive privacy and link pregnancy to other central human expressions of flourishing.

Indeed the central tenet of reproductive freedom is the fairly obvious fact that the reproductive life is central to self-identity, flourishing, and free expression more generally for individuals and families. While marriage is highly regulated, as are numerous sexual practices, no license is required for childbearing.

Because families and individuals have such broad freedoms in making children, advocates of reproductive freedom have maintained that it would be inappropriate, even discriminatory, to apply special restrictions to those who are infertile. Why ought the infertile person to be forced to undergo special screening prior to pregnancy when individuals whose reproductive capacity is intact can initiate pregnancy in the most unorthodox ways imaginable without fear of social scrutiny?

The argument against state interference in reproduction is a negative freedom.[2] Arguments for positive freedoms in reproduction, for entitlement to reproductive services, proceed apace. The standard of care for treatment of infertility is not obvious. While the clinical dimensions and etiology of a patient's infertility may be apparent, if the patient's underlying pathology cannot be treated (e.g., the testes repaired), it becomes unclear what the "cure" will be. Is the patient who has two children through in vitro fertilization cured? Which techniques, with what ends, should augment or substitute for reproductive capacity? Any answer to these questions will be textured by subjective considerations such as patients' ability to pay for services, the allocation of government resources to infertility research and treatment, and the technological limits of existing treatments.

Those who advocate the primary role of reproductive freedom in the human cloning debate point to the importance of allowing individuals and families to think for themselves about having children.[3] If the state allows couples to have children in squalor or single parent families, how can it reasonably proscribe human cloning as either unsafe or irresponsible? Some American scholars go so far as to argue that US restrictions on human cloning would violate the Americans with Disabilities Act, a law prohibiting discrimination against, in this case, and the infertile.

The pediatric model

On the opposite side of the human cloning fence are those who argue that human cloning would in some way harm children, and should be prevented in the interest of safety. The argument is made in the spirit of what we call the pediatric model, which emphasizes not the rights of procreators but the responsibility to care for those created.

In the twentieth century, healthcare for very young and very vulnerable children has become such a high priority as to rate inclusion in public health policy around the world. To see the enormous changes in the meaning and status of children one need only turn to the copious literature on the creation of childhood as an institution, which takes place during the twentieth century. Where one hundred years ago children made up a significant piece of the workforce, and infant mortality was a staggering 30-40 percent in some nations, today many parents can expect that their children will have access to comprehensive medical and educational resources. The identification of children's needs begins early, and among the very best-selling books in the world are guides to pregnancy and early childhood. Incredible amounts are spent on neonatal intensive care and high-risk obstetrical care, as the most vulnerable infants imaginable are kept alive even after extremely premature birth.

In ordinary terms, far from the tertiary care hospital, the pediatric metaphor is felt in public practice and policy about pregnancy and childhood. Parents in many nations come to know their child not as a child but as a fetus, with interests even early on in pregnancy. This can be mundane – an unnecessary ultrasound examination recorded on videotape to allow a mom to show the entire family her eight-week fetus. The presence of the fetus as an organism with interests has also presented extraordinary new problems. In *Griswold* the US Court ruled that the right to discontinue pregnancy does not include a concomitant right to willfully harm the fetus. In hospitals this can mean that women are assigned to social workers early in their pregnancy on the basis of their drug habits or other problems. They can choose to discontinue pregnancy without interference, but if they elect to bear the child in an environment that is dangerous to the child, steps may be taken – in advance – toward removing the future child at birth from the care of the mother.

Protecting children

The paradigm for such remarkable steps is the broad social consensus about the need to protect young and vulnerable children from dangers against which they cannot protect themselves. Parents who abuse or neglect children, who refuse to educate children, or who will not provide their children with medical care (such as vaccinations) can lose their parental roles. In this important sense, parenthood has always been both a responsibility and a privilege, rather than right, from the view of the pediatric model.

Arguments of the National Bioethics Advisory Commission and others that clinical human cloning should be prohibited have relied on the pediatric model. Two kinds of claims have been made, first that cloning would be physiologically unsafe for any human clone, and second that cloning would deprive a child of its identity or in other ways rob it of freedom. In the first case, it is clear that the claim is pediatric in character. Just as parents are forbidden from intentionally exposing their children to great, preventable risks, it is argued that parents ought not to expose future children to the sorts of hazards experienced by the first offspring in animal human cloning experiments. This duty obtains especially in early trials, when parents could have little or no confidence that their actions would be safe for resultant offspring.

In the second case, the argument of Dena Davis and others that children have "a right to an open future"[4] is also based on a social commitment to ensure that those who make children participate in certain pursuits taken by the community to be essential for the development of children. It is required in many nations that children be educated. The failure to provide children with clothing or a home safe from extreme violence is punishable throughout the world. In this regard it is feared that cloning might put children in an untenable family relationship or rob them of skills necessary for flourishing. The young clone might grow up with his or her progenitor as a "living" genetic test, knowing early on what is in store for his or her own future.

The litmus test for human cloning, from the pediatric perspective, is the interest of the clone. If it can be argued that the human child born through a new reproductive technology will be significantly imperiled in a preventable way, those who argue for the interests of the clone will hold that the procedure was unwarranted.

While arguments in the pediatric model seem very valuable to us, neither the pediatric nor reproductive rights model speaks to the question of how to regulate or debate human reproductive technology. Thus while we may agree with advocates of reproductive liberty that parents ought to have a wide berth in their sexual and reproductive choices, it is unclear how one would recognize any compelling interest that merits restricting that berth. And while we may agree that the cloning of humans does not take sufficient account of the interests of the clone, it is unclear how to prevent similar tragedies from taking place in low-tech parenthood, or how to regulate new reproductive technologies so that disaster is to be averted.

One significant impediment to dialog between those who argue for reproductive rights and those who argue for the interests of the child is the dilemma described by Derek Parfit. Because there is no child actually born at the time of the request for clinical human cloning, it at first seems odd to ask whether "the child" is well served by that procedure. One can only with difficulty protect the interests or rights of an organism that does not yet exist. Some even maintain that the debate about the interests of future generations must always be framed in terms of whether or not the future child would be better off never having existed. It is a seeming dilemma. However, there is one area of social policy where the gap between reproductive rights and the interests of children has been nicely bridged, resulting in significant consensus about how to protect children from dangerous situations.

The adoption model

Children have been adopted for thousands of years, and relationships between adoptive families and children have taken many forms and been articulated in many ways. The enormous institutional wisdom accumulated in what we call the adoption model can be very important for bridging the gap between reproductive liberty and pediatrics. The adoption model can move the debate about cloning and new reproductive technologies from its present, highly politicized rancor into a more constructive arena in which interdisciplinary and bipartisan consensus may be possible.

Parents who seek to adopt children are required, in virtually every nation, to seek prior approval from a regional authority or court. In many nations applicants are required to undergo psychological testing, home visits or other pre-screening. In most cases these pre-screens take place before a particular child has been identified for adoption; in many cases the pre-screen is independent and antecedent to the identification of a pregnant birth parent.

From the reproductive rights model, it might seem odd that such fulsome oversight is allowed. After all, fertile parents are not pre-screened before the state permits pregnancy. It could be argued that the screening of applicants for adoption is a manifest invasion of reproductive privacy and an incursion on the rights of parents to reproduce in the manner they desire. We might very well have converted adoption to the model of reproductive rights, following for example the US precedent of leaving surrogacy and egg and sperm donation to the marketplace. Why when we tolerate a virtual free market in all donor-assisted reproduction, with no pre-screen or judicial oversight, do we insist that adoption so closely monitored?

Best of both worlds

The answer is that adoption, in many respects, embodies the best features of both the reproductive rights and pediatric models. Adoption law is framed out of recognition that the adoption of a child is an unusual way to enter into a family, devoid of pregnancy and birth and textured by its own social and moral features. The adoption process cannot replace these elements of gestation and preparation for childbirth. However, in an important sense it gives communal imprimatur to the creation of a family, drawing on other social rituals for sealing a permanent and loving commitment (marriage).

The adoptive parents are not screened in search of perfect parents, only with the aim of determining whether or not this particular set of parents can provide some bare minimum features of parenthood that have been historically important in the adoption setting. In this respect the adoption judge is much like the divorce court judge.

When parents split up, a judge is in the unusual position of determining what sort of family is best for a particular child given some constellation of exigencies. What appears to us to be Solomon's wisdom embodied by such judges is actually the product of long-term study of human families in a particular communal context. While their decisions are imperfect, the ethical responsibility of the judge is identified with the representation that judge makes for the community and for the laws of the state or nation as they apply to adoption.

The adoption judge or magistrate is in an important sense a community historian for the dimensions of family, tracking some of the important features of the community so that they can be accounted for in matching parents and children. Parents who are not judged to be good candidates for adoption may plead their case, but are finally at the mercy of the community leaders.

The adoption model for human family making is predicated on several simple and profound assumptions. First, where unorthodox parenting arrangements (as in adoption or divorce) pose special challenges, the responsibility of the community to provide counsel and oversight is compelling. Second, where arrangements for parenting have not worked or are likely to present special problems, the court and community ought to be empowered to enact short- or long-term restrictions on certain kinds of family-making. Just as regional governments decide how marriage will work, who may inherit, and what kinds of schools provide a sufficient education, the family courts have a quite proper jurisdiction in prohibiting certain kinds of family relationships (e.g., incest, cloning, and polygamy). Third, the formation of a family is both a deeply personal and profoundly social act. The interests of children who are adopted or made through new reproductive technologies are best served when a spirit of openness and honesty about the meaning of the process is evident.

It is already clear that we join dozens of other ethicists and scientists in favor of a short-term ban on clinical human cloning. The purpose of this paper however is to argue for a way in which human cloning restrictions might take shape. Our claim is that clinical human cloning might best be restricted and stopped through attention to the democratic process and through a singular aim at protecting the interests of the children who would thus be made.

The adoption model can be easily adapted to a variety of reproductive technologies.[5] Our purpose here is not to argue for specific policies. We have explicated the framing of the debate both about human cloning and reproductive technology more generally, holding that while new reproductive technology can be discussed in terms of either reproductive rights or pediatric interests, the two kinds of arguments can seem incommensurable. Adoption as a model integrates both the importance of the rights of parents and the importance of the interests of children, even those children who have not yet been born or even conceived.

Where unorthodox parenting and family-making is concerned, the community should draw on much richer metaphors than simple analysis of rights. The conflict between reproductive rights and interests of the child is deceptively simple, reflecting more general debates in society about the role of the state in personal life.

By contrast the making of children is as complex and confusing an area as exists in human inquiry and human life. In adoption, somehow consensus has been reached that children of new and unusual techniques merit special protection, but such protection ought not to be onerous for parents once the parental relationship is consecrated. Moreover, by applying the adoption model to the problem of human cloning, it becomes immediately clear how difficult it would be for any of the test cases described above to meet the high standards for use of such a risky technology.

Parents who present with requests that would either excessively stylize children or place them in harm's way ought not to not be allowed to proceed. In the short term this will doubtless mean that under an adoption model, sponsored by state or regional governments, cloning ought to be proscribed. At the same time, unlike other larger plans designed to restrict a broad swath of scientific research, the adoption model is a more limited endeavor whose scope is the making of families.

Case 21 Two Genetic Moms: High-Tech Trouble or Double the Love?

Everyone has a mother. Some children have biological mothers, some have stepmothers, some live with adopted moms and some have moms who donated eggs or carried them as embryos for other moms who would raise them. Some kids have moms who they know well, others have moms they don't know, and still others have moms they don't know exist (most parents don't tell children about the use of donor eggs).

Some children grow up without the presence of a mother. Some children grow up and find a long-lost biological mother. One day children may grow up and find long-lost egg donor moms. One day children may have many moms – a mom who donates an egg, a mom who carries the embryo and a third mom who raises the resulting child. It is anyone's guess who the "real" mom is in the twenty-first century. Nature and nurture both contribute to parenthood, and in a complicated world of new reproductive technology, there are more and more ways to be a parent.

Introducing the eggshell mom

Scientist Jamie Grifo of the New York University reproductive program announced that he has added a new mother to the mix: the egg-shell mother. Using a technique similar to that in Ian Wilmut's cloning of Dolly the sheep, Grifo transfers the DNA from one woman's egg into an egg that has been given by a donor and from which the DNA has been removed. He then fuses the new egg together, and fertilizes it with sperm of the first woman's choosing.

The woman who donates the "emptied" egg, into which the DNA of another woman is placed, gives the child mitochondrial DNA, as well as some other genetic information that is floating about. The bulk of the genetic information in the new egg, though, comes from the "DNA donor," who will likely be the mom that raises the child. So some child will have a couple of "genetic" moms to think about, and a whole new story to tell about how he or she came into the world.

The more options, the better?

I love my mom, but I wonder why we would want to make a child with two genetic mothers. The answer is that, until today, women whose eggs are damaged have had only a few options: have no children, adopt or use a donor's eggs. In none of these cases would the genetic information from the woman find its way into any children raised by that woman.

This is troubling for couples because many feel like the use of donor eggs or sperm is a kind of invasion of their intimate life; they planned to make children through sex and using someone else's eggs or sperm can almost feel like adultery. Other couples just want to continue their genetic bloodline, and feel that as long as they are spending so much money on assisted reproduction, they may as well get as close to a "natural" birth as possible.

For men, the use of donor sperm has all but been replaced by the technology of intracytoplasmic sperm injection, or ICSI, which takes sperm that cannot swim or penetrate the egg and injects them directly into the egg with a tiny needle. This lets them make a genetic contribution.

Through Grifo's technology, women with mitochondrial diseases and other problems in their eggs will now have the same opportunity, if they can afford it.

The problem is that there is no way to tell what will happen with the technology. Some ICSI studies suggest that there is a possibility that children made through that technology will either inherit their genetic father's infertility problem or have a new problem in intellectual development. While Grifo's group got approval from a local ethics board, no one has announced plans to study this new kind of family, or to look at the long-term safety effects of the technology for kids. With 18 ways to make a baby, as Grifo proclaims,[6] someone should be studying how these 18 ways of family creation impact parents, children, and their short- and long-term outcomes.

The "shadow" of a mom

It is difficult to say what the long-term issues are in any of these technologies, because there simply is no effort underway to study either their medical or social implications for society. Do women have a right to make a baby through two-woman reproduction in a test tube? Probably so. Do children of the future, made through such a technology, have a right to grow up in a society that has prepared for their birth? Definitely.

I wouldn't want to be the first child to grow up with the "shadow" of a mom, who contributed something to me but we don't know what that something is. Should I meet her? Does she owe me anything? What if her egg shell contains a predisposition to disease – can I sue her?

But then again, maybe it wouldn't be so bad to be mothered twice over. Only time will tell.

Case 22   Grave Robbing the Cradle

Baby Brandalyn was born to Gaby Vernoff, who loved her husband Bruce very, very much. The Vernoffs seemed to lose their chance to make a baby with Bruce's tragic death. But Gaby found a physician, a very special kind called an andrologist, who was willing to take the sperm from her husband's dead body and freeze it in nitrogen.

The wife wanted to make a baby right then and there, and asked her in-laws for their blessing. Mercifully the elder Vernoffs asked her to wait, and grieve, before she made decisions about having children, which she did. Everyone wanted to do the right thing.

Still, while there is every reason to believe that Bruce wanted to make children, there is no evidence he would have wanted to have a baby made after he was dead from parts taken out of his dead body.

Recent research at the University of Pennsylvania suggested that more than three hundred women have made this request of physicians after the death of their loved ones. And it is difficult to see how you would turn down a wife's request to dispose of her husband's body in any way she sees fit. If a wife wants to cremate the body of her husband, we oblige her. If she wants to take sperm, we should also oblige her request. Taking the sperm would not be acceptable if the woman were a girlfriend or just a passer-by (the Pennsylvania study even found one case where an infertile nurse wanted to use sperm from a patient!).

And it would not be acceptable to take sperm if the husband specifically forbade it in his will. But taking the sperm is one thing, and using it something entirely different.

A difficult case

The physician involved in the post-mortem sperm case, Dr. Cappy Rothman, is a world-renowned and kind scientist and clinician. He says that this woman has thought about her desire to make a baby and that this is the first case where it seemed acceptable. So without sanction from any professional organization and without consulting any ethics board or even the broad community, he took the next fateful step and helped Gaby get pregnant. He wasn't worried about the fact that there was no specific consent, because in his view this was a couple that really loved one another and the child will be the product of that love. He was headstrong, and again we are in the position of evaluating a technology in the limelight of a hard case.

It is one thing to wish the best for Brandalyn. We can all hope that this child will have a good and healthy life, and that the love shared by her parents will enrich her potential rather than entangle her in difficult personal issues. But the ethical problem here is clear.

An issue of consent

First, it is wrong to reproduce without consent. This is the rape rule, and it is a very helpful starting point for evaluating new technologies that give us the opportunity to make babies out of just about anybody at just about any time. It is fine for dying men to make sperm donations and for their wives to use it. It is fine to put it in your will that you want a child after you die. But no one is obligated to carry that child for you, and you ought not make that child after your death unless you really did intend to have it.

If we don't have rules like this, before long we will be cloning Abraham Lincoln, Wolfgang Amadeus Mozart, and just about every dead athlete who broke a record and seems to have "wanted children at one time or another." Controlling the dead body of the husband is one thing, but making a baby from it is another.

Think of the child as well. Brandalyn may not be called Frankenstein or the Phoenix, but she will certainly be in line for some counseling. The question for infertility specialists is about responsible practice, and what it means to have a "good candidate" for a fertility procedure.

A good candidate for post-mortem sperm retrieval is one who gave consent. Period.

And even after consent, there should be some examination of the issues for each family. Will making this baby mean the wife can never remarry? Will it prolong the grieving process or even prolong denial of the death? How long should the family wait? Obviously no maverick doctor should be making this choice on his or her own.

Brandalyn is a baby with a very special future and a very unusual past. We wish her the best. But we ought not open the graveyard gates to in vitro fertilization until we have better rules.

Case 23   Baby Banking

Teenagers are not having babies as often now, and that is good news. In fact, teen pregnancy is in a near freefall, as more youth around the world are exposed to sex education and contraceptive methods. Still, far too many teens give birth to unwanted children and some resort to unbelievable tactics, even infanticide, to avoid raising them. Now, a German clinic has taken a radical approach to saving the children no one wants.

In 1997, the world followed in horror the case of a teen couple in Delaware who left their live newborn baby in a hotel dumpster. Since then, we have heard case after case in which kids have gone to extreme lengths to avoid letting the world know that they were pregnant. A New Jersey teen left her infant in a high school bathroom, only to return to the gymnasium for the remainder of her prom dance. In Germany, one teen couple dropped their newborn from a ski gondola, hoping to hide their mistake forever in a dying crevasse. Studies estimate that as many as 100 babies born to teenage mothers are abandoned each year. It is terrible.

Germany has a bright idea about how to stop the problem of teenagers who kill their infant children. It is called Operation Foundling and it isn't especially palatable. Think drive-through window. At a large German hospital and adoption center, a special depository was established this month so that those who wish to abandon their infant, anonymously, can do so in a way that maximizes the chance that the child will live and find parents who will care for it.

In one sense it is a touching and imaginative idea: offer those who feel they have no hope – teens with a terrible secret – a chance at redemption without penalty. In another sense the baby depository experiment just points to how horrific our social debate about adoption, abortion, and birth control has become.

But the Germans aren't the only ones who have developed ways to prevent baby-dumping. Texas was first US state to pass "safe-haven" legislation with multiple states quickly following suit including Illinois, New York, and Missouri. These laws, which do not guarantee anonymity or immunity, allow women who give up their unharmed babies voluntarily within a month of delivery and to use their actions as defense against prosecution for child abandonment.

Children should not have sex. But when they do, and when a 17-year-old's mistake becomes potential homicide, we need to have more to offer our children than morning-after pills, quick-fix abortions, and drive-through baby depositories. It is simply unacceptable that our teenage children believe it is better to kill an infant than to suffer the reproach of their parents.

We need to talk, as a society and in our religious and social gatherings, about how to declare war on infanticide. If illicit drugs merit a billion-dollar war and a czar, our government can spare a few dollars to make sure that our world's teenagers know that they have a choice when sex leads to pregnancy.

If the kids kill their children because they fear the stigma of teenage pregnancy and adoption, they have only us to blame. No deposit, no return.

Case 24   Cash Strapped American Fertility Docs Cry Out for Mercy

In 2005, *New York Times* news service spread this story all over the place:

> A bride at 49, Kathryn Butuceanu longed for children. But at her age, her best hope lay in fertility clinics and an egg donor, a quest she soon found could easily cost up to $72,000 for repeated tries. That figure seemed like a

deal breaker. Ms. Butuceanu (pronounced boo-tuh-CHAH-noo), an administrator at the College of William and Mary in Williamsburg, Va., and her husband, Cornel, a doctoral student, lived on about $55,000 a year.

But help came through a call to Dr. Sanford Rosenberg, a fertility specialist in Richmond, Va., who had started a program capitalizing on lower medical costs overseas. By using an egg donor from Romania and having the eggs fertilized in Bucharest and shipped back to the United States, the Butuceanus cut their costs to $18,000, including enough fertilized eggs for repeated efforts.

Yes, Romania. Paradise for late-life birth and, it appears, for egg donation. The article discusses a term that is heard more and more over drinks at the American Society for Reproductive Medicine (ASRM) conference: "fertility tourism," in which a patient can get a vacation in a tropical wonderland and infertility treatment (IVF – a full cycle) for the price of IVF alone in the United States. Or to put it more pointedly, eggs, medication, and medical care for IVF cost a fraction of the US price when purchased in developing nations.

The best thing about this article is the position that IVF docs take on the matter. Guess what they worry about? A lack of regulation overseas. You couldn't write comedy that good. Here are the practitioners of probably the least regulated field in all of American medicine, raising . . . substantive concerns about regulation of overseas clinics, genetic testing, standards for egg donors and language barriers, not to mention the difficulty in comparing pregnancy rates in American clinics with those abroad.

But wait it gets much much better. According to Sean Tipton, spokesman for the American Society for Reproductive Medicine, the cost of fertility medicine abroad is lower – in part – because of a lack of "research involving human embryos" there. Boy howdy does the average IVF clinic here do a lot of expensive research! Somebody remind me – how long was it before anyone in IVF conducted and published any kind of serious study on the effects of ovarian hyper stimulation medications on women's health? I forget. Two to three decades?

But there are all those expensive studies on outcomes for IVF – you know, studies about how IVF affects families. Oh, wait, that's right, those were almost all done in other countries. Hmm. Well, anyway, there must be some reasonable explanation as to why IVF costs a fortune here. It can't just be a seller's market. Can it?

Then of course, there is the flip-side of "fertility tourism" which has more recently resulted in foreign pregnant women showing up on our shores. Why? Quite simply, to give birth to an American citizen and then return home with a child who can have for the rest of his or her life the privileges of dual citizenship and being able to chant "USA! USA!" during the Olympics. Yes, it is true – despite our crumbling healthcare system and our obstetricians and gynecologists being litigated to within an inch of their subspecialty's life – women from around the world are giving American baby doctors big business. And for the price of two first-class plane tickets and a birth in a private suite (say $40,000), their child can have citizenship for life. Not a bad deal, I'd say. Not entirely ethical either though.

Notes and References

1. McGee makes this argument in *The Perfect Baby: A Pragmatic Approach to Genetics* (New York: Rowman & Littlefield, 1997), epilogue; it has been made by Wilmut and others as well.
2. Cf., Arthur Caplan, *Am I My Brother's Keeper* (Indianapolis: Indiana University Press, 1998).
3. See especially Lee Silver, *The Lives to Come* (New York: Avon Books, 1998) and Greg Pence, *Who's Afraid of Human Cloning* (New York: Rowman & Littlefield, 1998).
4. Dena Davis, *The Right to an Open Future*, Hastings Center Report, March–April 1997, pp. 34-40.
5. See, e.g., Glenn McGee and Daniel McGee, "Nuclear Meltdown: Ethics of the Need to Transfer Genes," *Politics and the Life Sciences*, March 1998, pp. 72-6.
6. Accessed at: www.pbs.org/wgbh/nova/baby/18ways.html.

Caution Five

Don't Sweat the Nano-Sized Stuff

Case 25 "Nanoethics": The ELSI of Twenty-First-Century Bioethics?

$42.6 million.

That is how much money is spent each year on ethical, legal and social research in nanotechnology by the US federal government.

In one year.

Have we moved to the era of genetics to the nanoscale age and I somehow missed it?

The age of the code of codes

Let's put that figure in perspective. Altogether – all included – the whole kit and caboodle – of ethical, legal, and social issues (ELSI) research dollars spent by the NHGRI (national human genome research institute) of NIH from the beginning of the ELSI program until 2003 totaled $125 million. Now NHGRI estimates to spend a paltry than $18 million per year on ELSI. This was famously described by Art Caplan as the "full employment act for bioethics," because it resulted in the hiring of dozens of new people to work in bioethics in institutions around the country: philosophers, doctors, lawyers, social and natural scientists, public health people, religion faculty … lots and lots of people who otherwise might have had little time or access to work on ethical, legal or social issues surrounding what at the time seemed like the most important new frontier in science and medicine.

There are plenty of critics of ELSI. I'm not one of them. I frankly think that the ELSI group has done an extraordinary job of accommodating

Bioethics for Beginners: 60 Cases and Cautions from the Moral Frontier of Healthcare,
First Edition. Glenn McGee.
© 2012 John Wiley & Sons, Ltd. Published 2012 by John Wiley & Sons, Ltd.

new methodologies – who would ever have funded a philosopher to study genetics prior to the genome project? As well as taking some important risks on studies that could very well have reflected poorly on efforts of the genome project itself: mapping of the genes of indigenous peoples, the impact of gene banking on members of disadvantaged groups, investigation of genes for "criminal tendencies." ELSI put bioethics to work and if it had not come into existence, bioethics as we know it today would probably not exist. We would still be reading about how "medicine saved the life of ethics."

Some folks who hate ELSI argue that it has made mercenaries out of philosophers and social scientists, that people followed the money. Others argue that research that might otherwise have been subtle or methodologically slower (more ethnographic studies published in books) was suddenly and woefully altered by the lure of filthy lucre.

But seriously, nobody ever got rich from ELSI money. And, of course, that isn't the way paradigm shifts work. Young investigators had to beg and plead dissertation directors to let them "bet their careers" on dissertations in genetics and society. Trust me.

The real story is more subtle. People whose interests were compatible with ELSI funding were able to do the sort of work they wanted to do by participating in endeavors that ELSI could reasonably fund – or merely by finding a way to work in places that were able to get ELSI funding from the genome project.

University bioethics centers, in many places, became plausible targets for money even beyond the ELSI grants because a viable argument could be made that indirect costs from ELSI grants would sustain the efforts not only of ELSI grantees but of ethics committee chairs, research ethics people, a real faculty to teach medical ethics, etc. And indirect costs – half again the amount of the NIH ethics grant paid for lights and coffee and air conditioning.

The age of bioethics "hub cities"

But the genome project's agenda for ELSI has changed. First, there was the odd effort to do most ELSI research "internally" through groups run out of the ELSI program offices themselves. It was creative, but many wrote and argued that this was not a great success, and it angered just about everyone who had already said that the ELSI study sections were becoming inbred. Francis Collins, then head of NHGRI, as early as 2003, began to give interviews in which he would lay out the roadmap for a "new" ELSI[1]:

"We clearly need to continue this in the most vigorous way," Collins told [one interviewer]. But NHGRI will be more assertive in steering ELSI grantees toward specific subjects, he said. "We're going to shift our emphasis more in the direction of topics that we know we need people to work on. We're also considering funding centers for ELSI research, as opposed to individual investigators. "The point is to develop institutions with a critical mass of different disciplines.

Correct me if I am wrong, but my review of the ELSI budget at NIH suggests the almost total aggregation of ELSI dollars by a set of Centers for Excellence in ELSI Research, sort of "hubs" for ELSI research, which receive huge hunks of money to accomplish lots of different projects. They are all great, and each is led by a researcher with a long track record of good ELSI research and other service to NHGRI and to science itself.

The Case Western site has projects in family studies, community, enhancement, commercialization, etc. The Stanford site studies "new models of deliberative, interactive processes that integrate ELSI considerations into the design and conduct of genetic research," and features projects on genetics and autism, a documentary film program, bench side ethics etc. The Duke program focuses on intellectual property, and ethics in society. The University of Washington site aims at: assessing the clinical utility of genomics, looking at the uptake for and impact on underserved communities, training, etc.

Get the picture? NIH has basically created four huge think tanks in genomics.

In other words, Collins has I think it is fair to say grown somewhat tired of ELSI as a free-for-all with hundreds of investigators competing willy-nilly for grants of all kinds. And there are reasons why that is problematic. It means that even though there is some significant research funding available for ethics and genetics, it is perhaps a third of the amount available for nanotechnology and society, and the amount of the NHGRI ELSI money that is left to build the investigators spread across the field of bioethics is minuscule once you pay for the Centers of Excellence in ELSI Research (CEER) awards. And like other core grants of their kind, the CEER centers are expected to help their junior investigators write their own grants – the "R01 pump" model in which the big centers are responsible for – and at huge advantage for – helping the junior scholars in their program to suck up still more ELSI money in order to do still more research to make each CEER center still better at the objectives laid out in the roadmap. So if you are competing for the remaining ELSI money after the CEER checks are paid, you are probably going to be competing with someone amazing from a CEER center, and with zillions of other folks.

Funding in ELSI genomics can no longer save the life of bioethics

It is fair to say that for up and coming researchers in bioethics, ELSI money from NHGRI is no longer a viable support structure for a career, unless there is reason to believe that one can work in a CEER center. Having recently served as the US reviewer for the equivalent of the CEER centers in the UK, funded by the Economic and Social Research Council (ESRC) there, centers that receive double or triple the amount of support, I can tell you that those who are training in ethics and genetics in the United States better start looking for jobs at Cardiff, Exeter, Lancaster or Edinburgh than trying to persuade an American university that there is ELSI money sufficient to support a funded trajectory through tenure track.

Now comes the age of small

Every year, $42.6 million in funding for ELSI in nanotechnology. But what does this really mean? What sort of funding is available, and what would pursuing it entail? What kind of person would build a career around nanotechnology and bioethics? Would it look anything like the bioethics scholarship that has grown up around genetics?

Let's "follow the money": just about everyone knows about the big programs in nanotechnology at the National Science Foundation, each of which requires some ELSI work by those who are funded with the big science grants. But there are other sources of funding: Environmental Protection Agency, Office of Research and Development, and National Center for Education Research offer funding, for example.

And there are journals coming, books, and of course new groups. Just last week this group was announced, comprised of those who have worked in some way or other on ethical legal and social issues in this, um, field. Ray Kurzweil. James Hughes. Vivian Weil. And there are places that work hard on this stuff, like Davis Baird's group at South Carolina funded with $2.8 million to study all sorts of stuff.

I have spent enough time with nanoscientists to get it that this is an interesting area of work with implications for public health and for enhancement. But, oddly, the purveyors of scholarship about ethical issues in nanotechnology have been ultra skeptical about the idea of "nanoethics," and have in fact done a fair share of "ELSI bashing," even before Congress. Langdon Winner of the STS program at Rensselaer Polytechnic Institute, e.g., testified to the House Committee on Science that:

> Studies of this kind could be launched in a number of ways, including funding truly cross-disciplinary programs in universities to scope out key issues and policy alternatives. But I would not advise you to pass a Nano-ethicist Full Employment Act [emphasis mine], sponsoring the creation of a new profession. Although the new academic research in this area would be of some value, there is also a tendency for those who conduct research about the ethical dimensions of emerging technology to gravitate toward the more comfortable, even trivial questions involved, avoiding issues that might become a focus of conflict. The professional field of bioethics, for example, (which might become, alas, a model for nanoethics) has a great deal to say about many fascinating things, but people in this profession rarely say "no."[2]

Ouch. And Baird, we noted, himself says that nanotechnology folks should avoid calling on ethicists "to patch things up as best as they can after the fact," preferring instead "humanists" and social scientists. Commentator and original guru of the Department of Defense's Energy's ELSI program Michael Yesley disagrees, saying that bioethics is still in the mix for these guys. But he's wrong. The new nano ELSI people seem to be steering as clear of "bioethics" as they can.

Baird is smart, funny and nobody's fool but it is notable that to get at the nanotechnology issues he is aided considerably by the USC Nanocenter on his campus. Just like ELSI for genomics, the pride of place comes from proximity and funding; the "nSTS" group is nested right within the nanotechnology group itself. Nobody's arguing this is a bad thing, but it is hard to see how it counts as a move beyond cultivation of institutions in which "bioethicists can't say no," at least not on its surface. How long do you thing nSTS would be funded if they began to argue that USC nanotechnology is horrific? I just do not know. But neither does Baird.[3]

Or maybe that isn't right. It is hard to tell. The program at USC is the paradigm case. It has tons and tons of projects – educational, scholarly, artistic. It answers to NSF, who have discussed their efforts in detail here.

Is there a there there?

I'm still quite clueless about what it is exactly that nanotechnology means, or to be clearer the sufficient conditions are for a thing to be correctly classed as the product of nanotechnology in as much as that moniker is opposed to something else. I have begun to read voraciously in the nanoethics literature, yet I do not understand the necessary or sufficient conditions for an activity to be nanotechnology.

I am not sure what it means for a scholar to have the special set of skills and knowledge to study social, ethical and legal issues in nanotechnology; are there "special" issues in nanotechnology that require the analog to the medical knowledge that a clinical ethics consultant must have in order to understand what it is that doctors are fighting about at the bedside?

But it is clear from reading just the 10 percent or so of the dozens of blogs and hundreds of articles that cross my desk in this area that there are interesting social issues here, and that they deserve serious consideration, whether they are special or not. They are there and even if the money devoted to "nanoethics" becomes much like that devoted to ELSI in its formative years at NHGRI, it is easy to see that careers built around the early study of the very small could yield very big scholarship, and new ways of communicating with the public. Even if at the end of the day the work these people do isn't primarily about nanotechnology.

And it seems clear too that the crowd who do nanoscience are just at the beginning of the curve when it comes to understanding the risks associated with making utopian projections for the future of bionanotechnology – projections whose analog in gene therapy resulted in huge misconceptions among research subjects. Just look to South Korea to see what happens when people believe that technology is earth shaking long before it can even shake the building.

Case 26   The Devil and the Deep Blue Sea

with Summer Johnson McGee

Just because I am an ethicist does not mean I am opposed to making money, particularly when it comes with solid scientific discoveries that benefit human kind. The field of nanotechnology carries that promise. Unfortunately, many ecorestoration, environmentalist or "green movement" corporations are more concerned with greener wallets than a greener world.

Planktos is a for-profit ecorestoration company, based in San Francisco, which aims to restore damaged habitats. Its plan is to release "forest-sized areas" of nano-sized particles of zero-valent iron (ZVI) into the ocean, with the hope that plankton will take up that iron, engage in enhanced photosynthesis, consume greater quantities of carbon dioxide from the environment, and curb global warming.

Planktos is not the only group seeking to capitalize upon the convergence of the green movement. Green building, using the advances of nanotechnology, could make our houses better insulated, more brightly lit with less energy, more efficient in countless ways, or nearly indestructible. The Green Technology Forum, a research and advising firm on nanotechnology, released a report that lauded "how a single nanotech innovation is saving one company $2.6 million in energy costs and reducing their carbon dioxide emissions by 35 million pounds per year."

This all sounds great, but early findings about Planktos' technology have not produced encouraging results, and multiple prominent scientists and environmental groups have debunked or dismissed the company's claims. Planktos is promoting bad science, which gives good and important science, namely nanotechnology, a bad name.

What is troubling here is that nanotechnology, being embraced the world over as the panacea for all that ails the way our materials work or our drugs react in the body, is being utilized in ways that at the very least could be described as reckless or, at the worst, harmful to the public perception and the progress of these technologies. The long-term implications of releasing ZVI into the oceans are not known. How will the currents carry these particles? How long and to what effect will the iron affect plankton plumes? What kind of warnings do we put on the houses of people living with paints with nanoparticles in them or whose walls of their homes are made of nanocomposites? Could these nanocomposites become the asbestos or lead for the twenty-first century?

What is also troubling is that there is no single body or organization responsible for monitoring nanotechnologies in any given arena – public health, environmental health, or other areas. We have no idea what the standards for risk assessment in these arenas should be. No single group governs or determines this, nor is there consensus.

There are a couple schools of thought. One says leave it alone, given that we are regularly exposed to all kinds of nano-sized particles from foods, pollution, drugs, cosmetics, and others. Another approach emphasizes being "responsible," encouraging caution and thoughtfulness, but it never defines what "responsible" really means. Others espouse the "precautionary principle," stating that if there is the potential for harm to the environment or the public, the burden of proof is on the scientists to prove that the technology is safe.

I think there's something more subtle that must be addressed. We can't expect scientists alone to conduct "responsible" research, given that they tend to embrace technology, and therefore approach the question with a bias. Leaving it to companies who have an incentive to release the technology, and start turning profits, is also not the way to go. Consequently, ethicists and the general public must be engaged in discussions about which of the technologies will be developed, when and where they will be introduced, and how they will be evaluated for safety.

We need a pragmatic approach to thinking about these technologies, which falls somewhere between the Draconian rule of the precautionary principle and the free-love view of the Wild West nano-loving scientists. And I am quite confident that such a path does not take us toward a giant iron dump near the Galapagos, nor a nano-house.

Case 27   The Merging of Man and Machine

In 1966, 20th Century Fox took moviegoers (and Raquel Welch) on a *Fantastic Voyage*. In this cinematic barn burner a diplomat lay near death from a blood clot, until, through miraculous technologies, scientists shrank a 30-foot-long clot-busting metal ship to the size of a pin's head.

Just about every American over 30 shuddered and gasped as the miniature ship sailed through the bloodstream, encountering white blood cells that seemed as large as the Brobdingnagian giants confronted by Gulliver on his travels. The ship's crew narrowly avoids destruction and its heroes are restored to normal size.

It was a fantastic first step toward human dreams of shrinking medicine to microscopic size. Today on the movie screen we are entertained by even more dramatic stories of kids shrunk to the size of ants and microscopic machines sent to infect the world. But is it just fiction?

Microscopic machines

Scientists have begun to create microscopic machines out of the chemical compound DNA. For years DNA has been described as a building block of life, but for scientists working on "nanotechnology," DNA may be the key to a whole new kind of genetic engineering.

The goal is to make devices out of organic material. As computer equipment, surgical tools, and communications pipelines shrink ever smaller, the next step in engineering is to merge biological and mechanical molecules and compounds into really, really small machines. This will happen in lots of different ways, and it raises lots of new issues.

First, we are beginning to see life forms reduced to molecular codes. This means that in our lifetime, viruses and components of our own DNA are going to become a lot more portable. Today, the last samples of smallpox virus are locked away in a vault in Atlanta at the Centers for Disease Control and Prevention. Tomorrow, getting smallpox may be as simple as forwarding an e-mail attachment with the smallpox DNA code to a $10,000 DNA synthesizer.

The portability of DNA also means that where you once thought of your DNA as a part of your body, tomorrow the DNA from any of your cells might be used to make a cloned embryo or to make a big sack of cloned tissue for transplantation.

Mix-and-match

Is it ethical to move life around this way, playing mix-and-match with bits from different animals and species? Should we create entirely new kinds of life from the molecule up? Would it be wrong to build a bacterial life form that depended on a machine for survival, such as battery-acid-powered carpet-stain-removal bacteria? Or is that no more problematic than executing billions of little yeast molecules to make a barrel of beer or a loaf of bread?

Second, enhanced DNA and computers are more and more becoming parts of our bodies. Millions watch as Captain Picard and the crew of the starship *Enterprise* battle a genetically engineered race called The Borg, who are the ugliest possible combination of DNA with computers (with the exception, of course, of new Borg sex symbol, Seven of Nine).

The Borg aren't real, but human-machine integration isn't just fiction anymore. Teams at MIT, Xerox, and elsewhere are racing to connect you very closely to your cell phone and television. Within a few years, pacemakers and other medical devices will begin corresponding electronically with hospitals, physicians, and even insurance companies about the patients whom they "inhabit." Many aspects of our behavior will be monitored more closely, and we may even get insurance discounts if we agree to "show" what healthy people we are!

What's "normal"?

Ethical issues in merging with computers go beyond the "weird "factor into a whole new kind of problem: what happens if human beings are made from non-human parts? Is a baby made from cloned DNA, gestated in a bubble and connected to a cellular phone still human? The answer matters because it is no longer obvious what it means to call something or someone "normal" or a "person, "even in the world of medicine. That means it is getting harder and harder to figure out which advances in medicine are worth public research money and which ought to be mothballed.

Third, and most interesting, we are approaching the world of Fantastic Voyage. Experts in this new field of nanotechnology promise a world in which very small machines literally circulate within us, pursuing bad bacteria and viruses and dissolving cholesterol and lipids. It sounds great, if a little bit spooky, but it is still a long way away.

So should we spend taxpayer dollars on clot-busting machines to extend the average life span, or work to build other artificial devices much smaller – and more effective – than the artificial heart of the 1970s? It is a difficult decision but one that only our generation can make.

Saving Social Security takes on a whole new meaning in a world that works hard to keep people alive well into their hundredss, but connected to dozens of expensive little machines. As we prioritize about hunger, our status as a global power, and the future of medicine, many of the most troubling decisions will be very, very small.

Case 28   My Eye's on You

Picture-perfect vision, with lovely dark pupils and irises of any color you want. Who wouldn't want that? Every person who wears glasses or contact lenses, or who just has that classic wish of the pilot or bird watcher – to see just a little bit better, farther, or more clearly at night – or who, vanity of vanities, wants slightly brighter green eyes, would be delighted to hear that stem cell research is moving us closer to the day when eyes might be created in the lab and implantable.

Looming is the prospect of creating human eyes (or at the very least, central components of the eye) for the purposes of replacing, repairing, or regenerating unhealthy or damaged tissue. Scientists are finding pieces of the puzzle, those factors that control the generation of eyes.[4] As eye researcher Nicholas Dale of the University of Warwick told LiveScience, "If you knew all the genes, and how to turn them on, that you needed to make an eye, you could start with very early embryonic cells and turn on all the right genes and grow an eye in a dish."[5]

If you think growing an organ in a dish sounds like science fiction, think again.

In "Betting on Better Organs,"[6] you can read about a US biotech that's growing human bladders in a laboratory from a small snippet of cells. The eye is considerably more complex than the elastic bag that functions as a bladder, but there's a long history in eye regenerative medicine, by stem cell research standards.

Ten years ago, a group used autologous cells from two patients each with one eye damaged by alkali burns, and both showed "striking improvement" after two years of follow-up.[7] In 2004, Advanced Cell Technology reported it had generated the first retinal cells from human embryonic stem cells. More recently, researchers at the Medical College of Wisconsin have begun to work on the repair of the eye with stem cells – including partially restoring the vision (enough to be able to drive an automobile) in a maintenance engineer who was burned by sodium hydroxide. But before you throw away your glasses, note that the studies that isolate the signal that turns on the generation of entirely new eyes have been performed successfully only in tadpoles.

Naturally, the work on stem cell therapies in the eye is mostly clinical and offers hope for those with severe eye damage, blindness, macular degeneration, cataracts, and more. But why stop there? Scientists such as Jay and Maureen Neitz at the Medical College of Wisconsin have been experimenting to see the effects of giving humans the ability to see different amounts of color when looking around the world, from dichromatic to tetrachromatic vision to even infrared.

Imagine eyes that are even better in terms of mechanics or aesthetics than the best endowed pilot, sharpshooter, or actor. How far from therapy for cataracts is the use of a gene for night vision? Scientifically, perhaps not far, but what about ethically?

The answer hangs on how you view enhancement. Literally. There are those who oppose the improvement of human nature on the grounds that we ought not to play God, or engage in risky research with no clinical benefit. But we are a society that enhances vision all the time with optical devices, ranging from night-vision goggles to colored contact lenses. I find it difficult to believe that building these changes into the eye itself would be morally more problematic.

If such technologies are available, and the implantation and maintenance of "eyes from the dish" is safe and effective, I would argue we should not draw an arbitrary line between enhancement for eyes versus enhancement for any other aesthetic feature on the body (such as noses or breasts).

Each of us may well have to decide just how far we are willing to go in terms of enhancing our perception. But the vision of better vision is coming to fruition. I'd keep an eye on it.

Notes and References

1. T. Powledge, "Wither NHGRI?," *Genome Biology*, 2003, 4: spotlight-20030417-02. Accessed at: http://genomebiology.com/2003/4/4/spotlight-20030417-02.
2. Netfuture, "Technology and Human Responsibility," May 2003, 145. Accessed at: www.netfuture.org/2003/May2003_145.html.
3. To read more about Yesley and Baird, see http://blog.bioethics.net/2006/01/tiny-ethics.html.
4. K. Massé, S. Bhamra, R. Eason, N. Dale, and E. A. Jones, "Purine-mediated Signalling Triggers Eye Development," *Nature*, 2007, 449: 1058-62.
5. LiveScience, "Scientists Envision Growing Human Eyeballs," October 2007. Accessed at: www.livescience.com/4670-scientists-envision-growing-human-eyeballs.html.
6. A. McCook, "Betting on Better Organs," *The Scientist*, 2007, 21(12): 30.
7. G. Pellegrini, C. E. Traverso, A. T. Franzi, M. Zingirian, R. Cancedda, and M. De Luca, "Long-term Restoration of Damaged Corneal Surfaces with Autologous Cultivated Corneal Epithelium," *Lancet*, 1997, 34(9057): 990-3.

The State Will Protect Your Health Right Up Until It Doesn't

Case 29 Has the Spread of HPV Vaccine Marketing Conveyed Immunity to Common Sense?

with Summer Johnson McGee

Approximately 20 million men and women in the United States are infected with human papillomavirus (HPV). For those whose infections are not transient, genital warts are the least objectionable problems caused by several versions of this sneaky virus, comprised of more than 200 permutations. HPV accounts for at least 65 percent of cervical cancer cases. It has become a scourge for sexually active women killing hundreds of thousands worldwide, most in the developing world, and more than 3,000 in the United States each year.

You would think that developing and introducing a vaccine that could prevent a vast majority of uninfected women from contracting those strains of HPV most highly associated with cervical cancer would be a no-brainer. Ignore for a moment the ethical imperative to improve public health that governs biomedical science. From a strictly financial perspective, it is cheaper to prevent cancer than to treat it. Moreover, if the sale of such a vaccine resulted in mammoth savings in terms of the cost of treating cancer, and in rising stock prices for the tens of millions who hold pharmaceutical stock in their mutual fund retirement accounts, that wouldn't anger anyone either. But all of those health and financial benefits depend on the public's use of the vaccine, so another ethical principle is at stake: should corporations become part of the public health system when

Bioethics for Beginners: 60 Cases and Cautions from the Moral Frontier of Healthcare,
First Edition. Glenn McGee.

their interests are so conflicted, lobbying to make their interventions mandatory, for minors and without informed consent?

It is easy to see why Merck, makers of the vaccine Gardasil, has to fight to get its vaccine approved. Crusaders against premarital sex argued against the vaccine on the grounds that it would increase promiscuity. Crusaders whose attention is focused on the risks of vaccines more generally have argued for delay after delay, insisting that the safety of the vaccine cannot be determined at this time. In May 2007, the conservative group Judicial Watch surfaced three FDA reports of deaths of young patients who had recently taken the vaccine, and 1,637 other adverse events reported to the agency. The revelation hits Merck right where it hurts: the company, still reeling from the Vioxx scandal, has created with Gardasil what should be the safest vaccine ever made, but which now may pose significant risks.

But the really hard-hitting criticism of Merck is coming, not from conservatives, but from mainstream journalists and liberals who argue that the vaccine costs too much. The *New York Times, Wall Street Journal, Associated Press, Philadelphia Inquirer, Atlanta Journal-Constitution* and more have carried stories or editorials in the past year in which Merck is hammered for the fact that it is spending huge lobbying dollars to make the vaccine mandatory. Even those who strongly favor the vaccine, such as Dr. Joseph A. Bocchini, chairman of the committee on infectious diseases of the American Academy of Pediatrics, are stunned at the degree to which Merck has pushed its $400 vaccine as a mandatory measure, rather than opting to phase in the vaccine at lower cost and with measures for informed consent and tiered pricing.

Merck suffered mightily from the Vioxx scandal, but Gardasil isn't a blockbuster pain medication nor a lifestyle drug. Vaccines are not Viagra. We all know that vaccine development is not going to easily yield a blockbuster. We learned this with pandemic flu vaccination, as the world asked why no corporation had worked to protect the public against such a threat. It just isn't a sustainable business model. But can't Gardasil make money for Merck without this high price? They clearly did not think so. After plumbing the depths of the direct-to-consumer market with Gardasil, it quickly became clear that the only lucrative strategy for dispersion of this life-saving vaccine was to mix metaphors: on the one hand, Merck deployed and paid for a traveling PR effort of female legislators who proclaimed that Gardasil was an unadulterated boon for public health – at any cost. On the other hand, Merck has positioned itself as the Halliburton of cervical cancer – Gardasil has, critics say, become akin to the $1,000 toilet seats on military aircrafts. Merck also dispatched lobbying teams across Washington, but more notably into the offices of governors and leading legislators across the entire United States, to carry the message that the cure for cervical cancer will save money, but only after the premium of an incredibly expensive vaccine is paid up front. In short, pay now, save later.

If pharmaceutical companies are going to fund lobbying to improve public health, they also need to support public health. A pharmaceutical company that can set aside billions in case it had to pay out big settlements or spend tens of millions to lobby government officials to order mandatory inoculation, also can afford to cut the cost of the vaccine. And now that the Gardasil has been studied, licensed and is for sale for use in men as well, the company, who has just doubled its potential market, can afford to cut a break to those living in parts of the world where a costly vaccine means it's a non-existent vaccine.

In addition, just as pizza bearing cheerleader drug reps are a poor substitute for medical education, pharmaceutical company lobbying is a poor substitute for well-reasoned public health policymaking. Merck should fund public health science, education and services so that, for example, we can learn more about who needs the shot, how to price it, and how to build a healthy relationship between the government, the public, and corporate biomedicine.

Case 30   Is the New Cigarette a Smoking Gun?
Eclipse Unethical, Unregulated Research

Eclipse – the reduced-smoke cigarette that its maker claims may be safer for smokers – isn't a cigarette. It is unregulated research, a massive uncontrolled study using a sizeable chunk of the smoking population as subjects.

No battle between the government and industry compares to the still white-hot debate about tobacco. There may not be a person alive who remains unconvinced about the health dangers of smoking cigarettes: lung cancer, fetal abnormalities, emphysema, heart disease.

Every American city has been reorganized – in its restaurants, its airports, its parks – so that secondhand smoke is eliminated. One tobacco company stands to lose billions in a class-action lawsuit.

The snowball effects of tobacco litigation and bad publicity – ranging from an expose movie to a year-long Congressional attack on Joe Camel that left him without a hump to stand on – promise to leave lots of the remaining tobacco industry holding a bag full of expensive IOUs to the families of those who died during our nation's 200-year experiment with unregulated tobacco.

On the other hand, tobacco is still huge business. The entire states of Virginia and North Carolina, and more than a few of the finest institutions in the southeastern United States (anybody heard of Duke University?) depend, or were built, on tobacco money.

Laundered tobacco money pays the rent for literally millions of workers in an industry that has associations with chemical workers, farmers, and stockholders.

The data suggest that just as many kids are smoking today as in the 1950s. And while smoking and use of tobacco has decreased slightly, the warnings and lawsuits have done little to change the nation's drive for the calming yet stimulating effect of the drug nicotine. It is delivered in a convenient little package at every bar and restaurant in the land.

Big tobacco also won the Superbowl of health litigation when it convinced the Supreme Court that the US Food and Drug Administration does not have the power to regulate tobacco.

Enter Eclipse. After spending $20 billion on attempts to create a healthy or at least low-smoke cigarette that still "tastes good," R. J. Reynolds Tobacco Company announced that it was about to launch a massive campaign to market a new and experimental product that is, well, sort of like a cigarette.

When big tobacco says it is launching a large campaign, fasten your seatbelts. There will be online sales of the Eclipse. There will be big promises about how Eclipse can help you stop smoking, or cut your health risks if you switch but keep puffing.

There will be much flaunting of the fact that the cigarette industry feels it is really not regulated anymore. The Eclipse burns almost no tobacco, instead warming it through a heating device that is lit "just like" the tip of a cigarette. The warming of the tobacco delivers nicotine, but slightly less than a cigarette does, as the smoker sucks air through the device. Eclipse, Reynolds claims, is a healthy cigarette.

But this isn't a cigarette. It is unregulated research. Reynolds has made a colossal miscalculation. The Supreme Court ruled that cigarettes are not devices or drugs and are thus not subject to regulation by the FDA.

But if there ever was a device that is designed to deliver a drug, Eclipse is that device. Eager to trumpet its commitment to health, Reynolds points to dozens of safety studies on all manner of animals performed before the launch of Eclipse.

We all know how reliable the tobacco industry's studies have been. But even if the studies about Eclipse show that this new device is safer, or even a good tool to help smokers quit, the point is that it should have submitted its studies to the FDA before it marketed this new product.

The ethical issues in tobacco are myriad, but this is the most obviously unethical move by a tobacco company since the decision to shred files and threaten witnesses in the 1980s.

Eclipse is a massive uncontrolled study using a sizeable chunk of the smoking population as subjects. No public review board has approved the study of Eclipse, let alone its sale as an over-the-counter drug.

And by the time there are data about this device and its implications, millions upon millions of Eclipse devices will have been used. More important, the clever and expensive attempt of the tobacco industry to force whatever device they make into a wrapper that looks and to some extent acts like a cigarette is a disservice to the public and to policymakers.

Whether Eclipse is the next step in the development of a healthy tobacco, or the final chapter in the tobacco industry, the unethical conduct of R.J. Reynolds deserves some scrutiny.

RJR's choice of names for its new product is ironic – Eclipse, defined as "darkness caused by obscuring a planetary or solar object that produces light."

So, before you light up your first Eclipse, ask yourself – Exactly who is in the dark?

Case 31   "Universal" Healthcare: A Long Way Off

The scenario is all too common. A man in Houston – let's call him Ed – works as much as he can to support himself on pretty meager roofer's pay. He has never met his boss, but his foreman told him there is no company insurance plan. Like most Americans working 28.5 hours a week in a permanent part-time position, Ed earns too much to qualify for Medicaid, but too little to afford good health insurance.

Like most Americans, Ed didn't think a whole lot about healthcare when he voted. He didn't think about insurance at all. Until he got sick. Now, Ed is one of 9.3 million uninsured Texans who will attempt to battle their way into one of the few remaining public hospitals and clinics that will provide them with care.

These patients may spend four or five hours waiting in the lobby of a large Houston hospital, hoping that an anonymous person in a white coat will see them and will be able to interpret and treat their problems. When they leave, they will sign some papers about payment, and 70-80 percent of the cost of their visits will be absorbed by the hospital.

These patients may never be able to get a credit card or mortgage, and their physical and emotional condition will likely worsen. It is this phenomenon that has closed almost every public emergency room in the Houston area. It is these patients' dilemma that has increased the cost of care in major, federally funded research hospitals by more than 1,000 percent in five years.

And even with the passage of the Affordable Care Act (ACA) in 2010, which promises to close the gap in the uninsured in America from 50 million to under 25 million by 2019, it remains to be seen if so-called "accountable care organizations" are anything more than New Age HMOs, whether the Tea Party will successfully repeal the Act itself, or whether Americans will ever understand the ACA enough to take advantage of it.

An ounce of prevention ...

The ethical issues about how America provides healthcare are giving way to more pragmatic concerns. Even those who continue oppose "socialized" medicine (read: The Affordable Care Act) are beginning to see the effect of failing to treat a huge uninsured chunk of the population. The sick get sicker, their poor families get poorer, and the time and attention in hospitals is shifted from preventing disease to rescuing the refugees of our medical neglect. Worse, whole not-for-profit hospital systems have collapsed under the strain, putting tens of thousands out of work in 1998 alone.

Many politicians are banking that Americans without health insurance do not vote and are reading the polls to see if those who do vote care about healthcare for the uninsured. They are counting too on the great American rescue ethic: hospitals will always save the sickest among us when they can, regardless of insurance. Thanks EMTALA (Emergency Medical Treatment and Active Labor Act). But the safety net of insurance for all Americans is not really about charity, or providing the best care for the minority who lack it. The real issue is a pragmatic one: our hospitals and insurance schemes are collapsing under the weight of the rescue ethic, and as a consequence health insurance for most Americans will be more expensive and less comprehensive this year than last.

Allowing Ed to become sicker and sicker hurts everyone. An ounce of prevention really is cheaper than a pound of cure. How that ounce of prevention will be provided expands beyond Accountable Care Organizations (ACOs) and health insurance companies and self-insuring employers who provide nudges for quitting smoking or losing weight. This kind of prevention will require a radical shift in how we understand and implement healthcare, a shift that will require putting public health and preventive medicine at the forefront rather than as an afterthought.

Case 32   Newborn Screening with a Twist

As of August 2006, New York became the first government in the world to start screening for Krabbe disease. The testing, which is expensive, can turn up, if there aren't too many false negatives, in the 1 in 100,000 infants born with the early onset form of this autosomal recessive trait that results in terrible symptoms followed by death typically before age 2.

In addition to the low incidence of this condition and the cost of its testing, the third morally problematic aspect of newborn screening for Krabbe is that no effective treatment exists. In 2005, a group at Duke conducted an interesting experiment that involved destroying the bone marrow of the affected infants with chemo, then replacing it with hematopoietic stem cells intended as a bone marrow transplant. It has worked, they report, 20 times, as best they can tell. But it is incredibly risky. Recent research evaluating the efficacy of Krabbe screening in New York reported that of the 550,000 newborns tested since the New York law was passed, just 4 infants at high risk of early onset Krabbe were identified and only 2 families opted for treatment. One of those infants died of complications from the hematopoietic stem cell transplant.

New York passed no law nor created a program to pay to enroll children in the experimental protocol at Duke, which isn't free, though some claim that payment from insurance companies might be no problem. Either way, the expenditure of this level of resource on an extremely rare disease, and where the risk of mis-identifying an infant who really has late-onset Krabbe, is difficult to justify when 30 percent of our nation, including poor women and children who could be covered by Medicaid, has insufficient health insurance for far more common conditions.

So why did New York add Krabbe to its battery of newborn screening tests? One reason: special interest politics. Former Buffalo Bills quarterback Jim Kelly, whose son was diagnosed with the condition, successfully lobbied the New York legislature to include the test as part of its newborn screening program.

Since New York added newborn screening for Krabbe disease, Illinois and Missouri have followed suit. Similarly, these states have made no provision for access to treatment. Differentiating between the severity of the disease detected, its time of onset, and its incidence is essential if we are to use our public health resources wisely. In the case of Krabbe, we have failed to address these distinctions. This failure may come to the detriment of our youngest and most vulnerable population.

Case 33   HIV Testing Must Be Routine

Centers for Disease Control and Prevention (CDC) in Atlanta has let it be known that it is going to change its guidelines regarding testing Americans for HIV. First, in 2006, the CDC recommended that all healthcare workers be tested for HIV infection. In addition, it has recommended that doctors offer HIV testing to all of their patients as part of routine medical care. The change is long overdue. In fact, it does not go far enough.

The change toward routine testing for HIV – the human immunode-ficiency virus that causes AIDS – is raising some ethical eyebrows. Some are worried that the government will know exactly who is HIV positive. This fear is understandable. Since the passage of the Patriot Act, our government has had unprecedented power to snoop on all of us without warrants. Plus, our country's well-known antipathy toward homosexuals, as evidenced by its use of anti-gay rhetoric as a wedge issue in the 2004 presidential campaign against John Kerry, show that stigmatization related to HIV/AIDS remains strong.

Others fret that busy doctors will harass poor patients into consenting to testing. As Catherine Christeller of the Chicago Women's AIDS Project told the *Wall Street Journal*, "Women –particularly minority women – have a concern about abuses." What starts as an offer might quickly become an expectation.

And still others worry that when you have routine testing offered, it may not be long before your boss knows the results. At companies that run their own health clinics, the promise of privacy is not especially credible.

Testing for HIV has provoked worries like these for more than two decades. That is why there has been no required or routine testing for HIV except in a few states, such as New York, which test newborn babies.

HIV testing has certainly been encouraged for people in high risk groups – gay men, those who utilize intravenous drugs and heterosexuals who have multiple sexual partners or sex with people who do, such as prostitutes – but encouragement is all there has been.

In some states, including New York, a special informed consent form must be used before testing for HIV. One consent to test was not deemed enough. And special counseling has always been recommended for all HIV testing.

So why change the policy? Because things are not at all the same when it comes to AIDS and HIV.

There has been a rapid increase in the occurrence of HIV in younger people who may not be as willing to practice safe sex or for whom those messages sound unnecessary. HIV is also occurring at greater rates in women who do not know about their husbands' various activities – visiting prostitutes, engaging in gay sex or using intravenous drugs. These women don't think they are in a high risk group and thus don't get tested.

There are now drugs that really work against HIV, and the sooner they are used the better. Twenty years ago, a diagnosis of HIV meant almost certain death. Today, a diagnosis of HIV is hardly good news, but there is a very good chance that people who are infected can live for decades with good medical care.

Plus the reasons to fear HIV testing are far less than when the epidemic began. Our legal protections are greater. You are not likely to get fired or told you cannot rent an apartment because you are HIV positive. The dire social and economic consequences that once awaited anyone unfortunate enough to have HIV have greatly abated.

What we need is aggressive testing. People who don't know they are at risk need to get tested. People who might benefit from the latest drugs need to get diagnosed. People who might infect others need to know that they could do so and do something about it.

Having doctors routinely offer HIV testing to all patients is a nice first step. Just by taking it, some of the last vestiges of stigma will evaporate from a diagnosis of HIV. But we ought be moving toward requiring HIV testing before surgery, admission to college or giving birth. It is unlikely that people would be scared away from getting healthcare or entering college by such a requirement, and there is every chance that a few more lives might well be saved as a result.

Old public health policies die hard. Our policy about HIV testing is getting very old and out of date. We ought to let it die.

Case 34   Re-creating Flu: A Recipe for Disaster

Pandemic influenza, whether of the avian or swine variety, continues to dominate news headlines. And for good reason. These viruses are nasty little critters. Why then would a recipe for how to make a nastier version of it appear in a leading scientific journal where anyone, including some of our worst enemies, can find it?

How bad is the avian flu that raced around Asia and Europe a few years ago or the swine flu that spread around the globe? If you compare the impact of the avian flu on your lungs to the regular old strain of flu that appears each October through March, it takes your breath away.

Literally.

Avian flu releases 50 times as many infectious particles in the human lung as does an ordinary flu virus. If you wait 4 days, there are 35,000 times as many virus bits in a mouse lung infected with avian flu than are present in good old normal but nasty flu. In mice, 100 percent are dead a week after infection compared with a few deaths from other flu viruses.

When influenza first struck globally in 1918, it killed as many as 50 million people worldwide. Pandemic avian flu, were it to break out again, could kill just as many people, if not more. And even despite the very best efforts by the CDC and vaccine makers, we know that existing flu vaccine only protects against certain strains of seasonal and swine flu. The time required to make an effective vaccine can mean millions will get sick and die in the meantime, and we lack sufficient vaccine production to vaccinate everyone.

Prescription medicines like Tamiflu may not do much if you do get infected, and a naturally occurring strain of avian flu resistant to Tamiflu has already been discovered. About the best you can hope for is not to get infected, using something now defined in the literature as "social distancing." This is pretty difficult to pull off at a time when modern air travel means someone can be infected in Romania, Thailand, or Indonesia on a Monday and be standing next to you on a street corner by Tuesday.

Given this grim picture, you might imagine that the last thing scientists would try to do is to create this, or a similarly lethal bug in the lab. You would be wrong. A team of scientists recently announced in *Science* magazine they had re-created an artificial version of the original pandemic 1918 flu virus.

At a time when the war on pandemic flu is a top priority, why are scientists making a similar deadly virus in their labs?

One explanation is that, by building this bug, it may be possible to understand every bit of its genetic blueprint. That information could prove invaluable both in identifying any naturally occurring viruses and in developing a vaccine against avian flu.

However, it is not at all clear that the re-created virus is being kept in such secure confinement that a bioterrorist could not get his or her hands on it. Worse still, publishing the entire recipe for how to make a deadly virus gives every terrorist group and nut-ball outfit in the world the opportunity to try their hand at making the virus, too.

The state of the art in science is that scientists have only truly accomplished something when they prove it with publication in carefully peer-reviewed publications. Putting the virus out there for peers to judge was the logical next step along the path to understanding and controlling the machinery that fuels a potential pandemic.

People in the life sciences hate the idea of government meddling in their work. They believe the free exchange of information is the best defense against a nasty pathogen like avian flu, whether it gets here on an airplane or in a terrorist's bomb. But can we really be sure that every step has been taken to keep existing samples of flu secure? And does it really make any sense to publish the complete genetic blueprint for the virus where anyone can find it? Perhaps not.

A decade ago, the manipulation of deadly viruses could be restricted to a high-security vault, a hot-zone under lock and key. No one had anything to fear from a scientist's description of a virus. Today, however, the super-secret stores of deadly viruses have been reduced to a set of instructions, which might at some point become a cookbook for terrorists and other malcontents or amateurs.

At a time when there are no means to easily prevent the spread of pandemic flu and few effective means to treat anyone who gets infected with it, there is a need for much more accountability about who should be making this and similar organisms. And, we need to be especially vigilant about who they should be telling about how to make it.

Case 35 Pandemic Influenza Requires Trust in Government Healthcare

The message from scientists and public health agencies the world over is clear: It is only a matter of time until a pandemic influenza outbreak circles the globe. In an age of air travel there will be little advance notice of its impending arrival, this pandemic will likely kill millions. It is a time when Americans must believe that their health and safety is in the hands of those whom they can trust. But they don't.

Anyone who has watched the nightly news or read a newspaper article about pandemic influenza knows that no matter what we do, we will not have enough vaccine or pills to protect even a quarter of the American population any time soon. Let alone the world. Only two things can slow the spread of pandemic flu, and they are the scariest things in the armamentarium of medicine: quarantine and rationing.

Quarantine was pioneered in fourteenth-century Venice, where ships were required to wait offshore for 40 days to clear sailors of disease. During the 2003 SARS outbreak in Toronto, quarantine entered the twenty-first century: 45,000 people in that area were asked to remain in home quarantine for 10 days.

Luckily, Americans seem open to the idea of quarantine. The US Centers for Disease Control says that 85 percent of those whom they polled are willing to stay home and care for themselves or their families in a pandemic flu outbreak. More than half would be willing to limit contact with others for a month or more. Even better, they seem open to the idea of rationing. About half even said that they would be willing to wait months for a vaccine so that clinicians and other leaders could be vaccinated first.

But researchers at Harvard School of Public Health[1] have found people won't do any of this if it is called a "quarantine." That term calls to mind images of martial law patrolling the streets to protect the well from the sick and stigmatized.

The name isn't the only problem with public participation in preventative measures before and during a pandemic. Whether you call it, as some suggest, "community shielding," "social distancing," or neighborhood clustering, or for that matter, just a prolonged slumber party, the public will accept public intervention to prevent disease only if they trust the American healthcare system as well as their government.

And they don't.

Trust requires transparency. When public officials fail to reveal in the most public way the stark truth about the plans of cities, counties and states in a pandemic, it is a prescription for panic. Citizens of a country where those in one state have "Live Free or Die" on their license plates will not take kindly to being imprisoned in their homes unless those measures have been presented as part of a comprehensive strategy that takes their sacrifice of liberty into account for some higher good, such as saving their lives.

They would be much more willing to stay home with their families for a month to prevent the disease's spread if they trust those deputized by the national and state agencies that implement the directives of the Centers for Disease Control and the Department of Homeland Security – and if they are sure that they will not be left to rot while others receive better care.

For these same Americans, rationing is as terrifying as quarantine: If too few drugs, too few healthcare workers and terrible medical facilities plague our larger urban areas, imagine what could ensue. Cutting in line will be the least of our problems. Americans must believe that the questions about profit in the development and distribution of vaccines and anti-influenza drugs will fly out the window when the pandemic arrives.

American medical schools and medical associations must reinstill a strong sense of professionalism in medical students and healthcareworkers or they may not be there in the face of danger. The public has taken notice that more and more physicians have refused to work weekends or nights. What makes us think that they will work 24-hour days knee deep in highly contagious patients unless they have a strong sense of professional ethics and duty?

The only answer to these challenges is to build trust and inculcate responsibility. If people understand the rationale for quarantine and why some people must be vaccinated ahead of others, they are more likely to accept hard choices. Building trust means immediate public education, town meetings at which officials listen as well as talk and plans sensitive to local concerns. And it means that all healthcare workers, though many will arrive ready to serve, will have to be convinced of their civic duty to care for the sick in a time of crisis, even if it is at the expense of themselves or their loved ones.

Modern medical ethics has never been tested so dramatically. On the one hand, we had better have a government willing to move fast and yet one that will err on the side of caution. We need a better public health sentinel system to limit the pandemic's spread and a public ready to yield some liberties.

The policies under development are frightening and depend for success on public trust that isn't there. As a pandemic looms in the offing, the billions of dollars spent on surveillance, intervention and quarantine will neither stop a pandemic nor those who have it unless the public trusts those who will be kicking the military machinery of quarantine into place.

Case 36   A Hostile Environment for Environmental Protection Documents

Like most US agencies charged with the oversight of the public's health, the Environmental Protection Agency (EPA) relies on accumulated wisdom as it navigates new and varied problems. So imagine the information it stores at 27 libraries: books, journals, reports, and documents numbering in the millions. According to agency statistics, in 2005 EPA library staff fielded more than 134,000 database and reference questions and distributed tens of thousands of documents to researchers and the public. The library is the institutional memory of the EPA. Yet the EPA library shutdowns have depleted reference material that might be indispensable in an emergency.

Like most libraries, EPA libraries have not scanned most holdings into electronic format. So librarians and location- or specialty-specific repositories are important to the EPA and those who consume its information. You'd think that the agency responsible for, say, all clinical information on the effects of pesticides would do anything to keep those systems of information fully operational and to modernize. But in fact, the greatest environmental disaster of this decade may be the amnesia that the White House and EPA seem hell-bent on causing.

In February of 2006, the White House proposed cutting $2 million of the $2.5 million budget for EPA libraries. It is a huge cut to the libraries, but a blip against the $8 billion EPA budget. Incredibly, EPA did not wait for the budget to be approved, but instead began decimating libraries and trashing materials including at three regional libraries, a library for research on the effects and properties of chemicals, and its headquarters.

Senators Barbara Boxer (D, Calif.) and Frank Lautenberg (D, N.J.) and associations representing thousands of EPA scientists, engineers and other staff cried foul, pointing to the fact that EPA shutdowns depleted reference materials that might be indispensable in an emergency. In the EPA's library, for example, are at least 50,000 one-of-a-kind primary source documents. The EPA's own Office of Enforcement and Compliance Assurance (OECA), said last year that the agency has failed to adequately maintain critical information and accessibility. OECA "fears that dispersal of [the libraries' information important to specific regions ... and unique data on industrial processes and analytical methods] without proper tracking and access could undercut rulemaking and the ability to substantiate and support findings, determinations and guidance."[2]

Representatives Henry Waxman (D, Calif.), Bart Gordon (D, Tenn.), and John Dingell (D, Mich.), called on EPA Administrator Steve Johnson to stop the process and the General Accounting Office to investigate. EPA says it has stopped. But it has failed to make available a good plan for access to stored materials. They just disappear. How? I find an image from the 1981 film *Raiders of the Lost Ark* helpful: scientist Indiana Jones is told by bureaucrats that the ark is being examined by "top people" and will be available later. The camera fades to the ark fading into a massive warehouse. EPA ought not to become a shell, or shill, manipulating its identity or even recreating itself as every administration relegates to "top people" the documents that are necessary to ensure public health.

Some have alleged that the EPA is shredding not just journals and documents, but files that may specifically damage the agency. No one has provided any proof of that yet, but if it turns out to be true, it may deserve a column of its own. My point is more mundane, but perhaps just as important. We just have to look to history to see the effect of destroyed libraries. Take the loss of the Library of Alexandria, founded in the third century BC, to fires likely set by scoundrel politicians.

The Alexandria loss became iconic when Carl Sagan created a digital recreation of the library for the famed television program *Cosmos*, and strolled through it to illustrate how political attacks on science can have a vast, pernicious effect on scientific progress. Data about pesticides isn't on papyrus scrolls, but the destruction of EPA's library system might have as much effect on our ability to monitor the environment as the burning of the 500,000 scrolls in Egypt.

The EPA, in the midst of an inspection of its clinical trials by a committee that includes ethicists, can ill-afford to lose its memory. And it owes all of those human subjects and the public access to relevant records. It is a hostile environment. Congress can spare $2 million to repair it.

Case 37   To Quarantine or Not to Quarantine, Is That the Question?

In 2007, one man single-handedly exposed the fact that the US public health system doesn't always do its job. Infected with a deadly drug-resistant strain of tuberculosis, Andrew Speaker traveled to several countries, exposing more than 600 people on two flights, even though a scan of his passport brought up a warning to keep him in custody and contact health authorities.

One could argue that it's the public health system's fault that he developed multi drug-resistant tuberculosis (XDR-TB) in the first place. TB becomes resistant to antibiotics when improperly treated, and MXDR-TB is resistant to at least two main first-line drugs. If we thoroughly treated TB in its less deadly-form, the US Centers for Disease Control and Prevention wouldn't have had to institute its first federal quarantine in since 1963.

It is clear that our current system of directly observed tuberculosis therapy, in which healthcare workers watch patients take their TB medicine, may not sufficiently ensure that people receive appropriate treatment and cure. Although the incidence of TB in the United States reached its lowest point in 2010 (3.9 cases per 100,000), that same year, the rate of decrease was down significantly from 2009. Moreover, the number of people with drug-resistant strains of TB remained steady at approximately 1 percent of cases, but each year at least one XDR-TB case emerges.

But Andrew Speaker has not been the only person to alert us to our inability to control infectious disease in the United States In February 2011, a New Mexican woman with an active case of the measles traveled through four US airports, potentially infecting hundreds on the airplanes in which she flew. Like Speaker, who had been non-compliant with treating his TB, this woman had refused to be inoculated with MMR (Measles, Mumps, Rubella) vaccine. There was little that could be done once this "Typhoid Mary" had been identified except to quarantine her, except, at least one ethicist has argued,to sue her for damages.

Infectious disease control has not significantly advanced since the fourteenth century, when quarantine was the preferred method for controlling the spread of plague in Europe. Now, the meaning of quarantine is often less specific than it was in Italian harbors seven centuries ago. During recent drills for combating bioterrorism, US officials have confusingly used the word to describe a number of different containment strategies, including limiting travel, restricting public gatherings, and isolating infected people.

Even now, the rules about quarantine don't seem crystal clear. The CDC ultimately decided that Speaker had a quarantine-worthy strain, and local officials told him not to travel with TB. According to the CDC, the only enforcement in place was a "covenant of trust," which obviously wasn't enough.

So what should local health officials, or the federal government, have done differently? Quarantining people against their will could easily be interpreted as a violation of civil liberties. (In an interesting twist, Speaker is a personal injury lawyer, and his father-in-law is a prominent TB researcher at the CDC.)

History contains many incidents during which imposing quarantine went horribly wrong. In the late nineteenth century, the New York Port Authority placed ships traveling from regions hit with a cholera outbreak under quarantine, but it did not care for all passengers equally, and the disease spread rapidly among the poor. In 1900, in response to a plague outbreak, officials established a quarantine on only Chinese residences and businesses in San Francisco, causing severe economic damage to the community. A federal court later ruled that the quarantine was unconstitutional.

So, officials didn't violate Andrew Speaker's or the New Mexico woman's liberties, but what about the interests of all the airplane passengers who spent hours with them, and now need to go through the trouble of getting tested and protecting their family and friends?

There is more to public health ethics than protecting civil liberties. We have not yet, as a society, thought through collectively how we want to handle, from a public policy perspective, events that are highly unlikely (the CDC recorded less than 50 cases of XDR-TB from 1993 to 2006), yet could be catastrophic. Alternatively, there also must be public health strategies for what are likely to be increasing outbreaks of diseases like measles and mumps as greater numbers of individuals abstain from vaccination. We will have to ask ourselves whose rights and interests come first during public health challenges: the non-compliant and infectious or those of the general public? That question, still unanswered, is as old as quarantine itself.

Notes and References

1. Accessed at: http://content.healthaffairs.org/cgi/content/abstract/25/2/w15.
2. Letter from Senator Barbara Boxer, November 3, 2006: "Boxer Leads Senators in Call for Restored Access to Epa Libraries." Accessed at: http://www.yubanet.com/cgi-bin/artman/exec/view.cgi/22/45080.

Caution Seven

"Do No Harm" Has Become "Care for Yourself"

Case 38   Medicine Is Not a Steel Mill

Imagine the worst working conditions: child labor, no medical coverage and appalling disregard for the physical safety of employees. Imagine a tyrant boss who can fire you at a moment's notice, leaving you destitute and with no other jobs in sight. Imagine coal dust or iron flakes or dirty chemicals so thick you cannot avoid touching and breathing them every day. If you can't imagine that world, you have labor unions to thank.

Even those who hate organized labor unions acknowledge that they played a critical role in protecting vulnerable workers from predatory bosses. And they built communities too. Workers with terrible and pointless jobs stopped being serfs and began to think of themselves as partners.

Again, great stuff and an important part of our history.

Only guess who wants a union now? Another group who has been abused? An impoverished mill town in North Dakota?

No, it is the best paid profession in America, the group with the most prestige and public standing. Why would doctors want a labor union? It is simple math.

Before managed care, physicians were paid more to do more, and all the fat in the healthcare system went to physicians' salaries – to the tune of an average 10 to 15 percent salary increase per year.

Now, with nurse practitioners doing everything but surgery for roughly 75 percent of the cost of a physician, and with managed care companies demanding that physicians be more frugal, your doctor's salary is, well, stagnant.

Bioethics for Beginners: 60 Cases and Cautions from the Moral Frontier of Healthcare, First Edition. Glenn McGee.
© 2012 John Wiley & Sons, Ltd. Published 2012 by John Wiley & Sons, Ltd.

He or she isn't breathing coal dust, and you can bet that medical coverage isn't a problem. Medicine is not a steel mill. There is no big bad boss.

The battle against managed care grows tiresome. We all agree that office visits should be a little longer and that patients are entitled to air, quality treatment. Managed care companies can do a much better job, and they had better recognize that they are accountable for what they do and don't do to patients.

But that isn't what the American Medical Association's endorsement of labor unions is about. A labor union doesn't represent you and me. It represents our physicians.

And with the highest physicians' salaries in the world, it is really really tough to feel sorry for these new American "enemies of management." It is time to get focused on the real ethical issue: making sure patients are treated as well as their physicians.

Case 39   Does Your Doctor Have Skeletons? Good Luck Finding Them

Everyone makes mistakes. Pilots forget to file flight plans, bus drivers forget to use a turn signal, and teachers forget their lesson plans. Just as you might suspect, medical mistakes happen too. What you might not suspect is how often they occur and how deadly they can be. Recent studies suggest that medical mistakes cause more deaths than gun violence, bus crashes, and airplane accidents combined.

And you might be surprised at what happens when physicians make mistakes. In the world of medical ethics, there is an unkind truism: When clinicians make mistakes, they begin shredding papers, coaching colleagues and generally doing just about everything they can to make things worse for everyone involved.

Whether it is the sponge left in the abdomen during surgery, the accidentally transposed numbers in a dose of medicine or even the amputation of the wrong limb, medical mistakes are scary. And they can have a big impact on patients.

Lately, that impact has been on patient trust. Polls show that patients are increasingly unsure about their caregivers' many conflicts of interest: If an HMO rewards doctors who refer fewer patients to specialists, for example, would a physician in that plan defer a referral longer than is prudent? Many are unsure.

Trust in physicians has not been helped by scandal after scandal in which all parts of the healthcare system seem to be colluding in an effort to hide medical mistakes and prevent costly lawsuits. Some 95 percent of doctors say they personally have witnessed a serious medical error, according to a survey released last month, yet most go unreported.

And now, a new federal study concludes that despite clear reporting requirements, 84 percent of HMOs and 60 percent of hospitals have not reported a single medical error in the past decade.

Protecting yourself

So what do you need to know about medical mistakes and how can you protect yourself? The first thing to understand is that medical mistakes are more complicated than figuring out that a physician or nurse goofed.

Stark statistics that 45,000 to 100,000[1] Americans die each year of medical mistakes seem to point the finger at individual caregivers. Indeed, it makes sense to hold physicians responsible if they hide mistakes that future patients should know about.

But the cause of the mistake is almost always bigger than the individual physician or nurse involved. If the unspoken – or perhaps even the spoken – word at many HMOs and institutions is that the physician is allowed only 8 or 10 minutes per patient, or is not allowed any staff support, or cannot refer the patient out for specialized care, then part of the blame goes to the system that the physician participates in.

If the hospital where the physician works cannot afford to employ nurses instead of untrained health "helpers," can we really hold the physician solely responsible when there is no longer anyone to catch a mistake in his or her written prescription?

Medical mistakes have spawned a whole new kind of "protect yourself" movement in American healthcare, and it is easy to see why you would want to make sure that your kids' pediatrician hasn't killed anyone lately.

In the Internet age you will not be surprised to learn that the Federation of State Medical Boards collects information on disciplinary actions against doctors across the country, which you can access for $9.95 at www.docinfo.org, or that more than a dozen other web sites purport to let you check out, for a fee, any medical mistakes your clinician may have made.

But before you plug "Dr. Smith" into "doeshehurtpatients.com," consider this: Such sites may tell you less about what kind of doctor he is than you think.

The real question you need an answer for is this: Can you trust your clinician? And the only way to answer that question is to pay for a little extra office time so you can get to know him. Or if possible, do a little detective work by asking other patients how they feel about him.

Numbers about skeletons in the closet can be deceiving. Ultimately what you want to know is not "Did he make a mistake?" but "If he makes a mistake, what will he do to fix it?"

If you think the answer is "duck and cover," find a new doctor.

Case 40 Medicine's Dirty Laundry

Most of us know almost nothing about Florence Nightingale. The hero of nurses around the world, she is remembered by most as the "first nurse," or as the patron saint for caring for the sick. What is amazing about Florence Nightingale, though, isn't the fact that she was among the first well-educated nurses, or that she cared so deeply for so many of the sick. Truth be told, nurses were caring for patients hundreds of years before she was born, to a very wealthy family, in 1820. Florence Nightingale did turn medicine on its head, though, and started a real revolution. And we are overdue for another one just like hers.

In 1853, a 33-year-old Nightingale received a letter from a friend in the British government in London begging her to quit her quiet job managing a small nursing home for nannies. Britain was involved in the terrible Crimean War against Russia, and Florence's friend asked her to come to the desolate lands between Turkey and Russia and assist the British government's emergency field hospitals.

What she found in the field hospitals stunned her. Surgeons were working day and night to repair horrendous wounds from 1850s weapons. But most of the death and suffering did not come from the actual war wounds. The men of the Crimean War died of poorly designed hospitals, bad sanitation, lack of staff, bad nutrition, lack of laundry, and countless other problems that came not from bullets but from bullheaded administration and a lack of foresight.

Sick barracks

The singular accomplishment of Nightingale was to turn the attention of those who were fighting the war away from how many soldiers died from bullets to how many soldiers died from what she called "sick barracks," conditions so bad in the field that no soldier could have fought the war.

She wrote letter after letter in Crimea and throughout her life to turn the attention of the British Parliament away from simplistic, magic-bullet approaches to medicine. Every step of the way Nightingale had to fight a hard battle against those who argued that doctors, not clean laundry and ventilation, keep us healthy. She would finally lose her highest priority battle: to close most hospitals in Britain, treating as many people at home as possible.

We have come a long way since the Crimean War. We live longer and better lives. But the most important lesson of Florence Nightingale has been all but lost in our visions of the future. Looking at many recent media reports on predictions for the next century, what you find is a pill for this and a pill for that. Pills will make us live longer, and look younger, and kill off every bad virus and thwart every cancer.

Guess what: That's what they thought in Rome, too. In the second and third centuries, there is every indication that the Romans believed that their century would see eternal life from new and revolutionary "pills," manufactured in the most careful way. Throughout their empire, Romans made a toast to their future medical success, raising a lead glass filled with water that came from their lead pipes.

The lesson of Nightingale is to pay attention to what really sustains human health, and put your energy into making sure that people have those basic, dull essentials. The most important studies of human populations and human health through the centuries show one irrefutable fact: the impact of public sanitation on public health is at least ten times more important than medicine – all of medicine – for sustaining health.

If all the hospitals in Chicago shut down for a week, there would be chaos and perhaps a thousand people would die. If the sanitation system of Chicago – trash and sewage treatment – shut down for a week, the entire city would be sick, and millions would quickly die.

Protecting the environment

Medicine is essential and its advances are amazing. But the most important part of health has nothing to do with medicine as we currently practice it. The most important part has to do with a healthy environment.

The city sewage systems around the world, and particularly in the United States, are aging and many are vulnerable to pollution, overflow from rain, and insufficient staff. Many of us work in "sick buildings," which recirculate almost 100 percent of the air and do little to filter out impurities.

Research from Australia has shown that adding a few ferns to your office won't filter out that danger. Formaldehyde (that "new car smell" found in almost all new carpet and plastic products in offices and many homes and cars) is a key pollutant that has been linked with many illnesses, and studies have shown that you would need to put a jungle in your office to counteract its effects.

Virtually everything we eat and buy is packaged in plastics that, some studies suggest, may have health effects in the long term. And, in the new millennium, we have begun to radically alter the way we feed ourselves, ranging from the ubiquitous powdered diet drink, to cereal bar "nutraceuticals" loaded with extra herbs and vitamins, to foods modified at the molecular level to cross vegetable with animal.

While most of us do not drink water from lead pipes, there is lead in your grandmother's fine china and in the paint on the walls of virtually every home built between 1930 to 1970.

It is an exciting time to be alive, and lots of people I talk to are hopeful that those alive today may manage to live an extra 20 or 30 years from the breakthroughs in medicine. But the simple math remains. Florence's math tells us that while we can spend billions to cure diseases with medical intervention, it would be infinitely more cost effective to spend half of that money on preventing disease through research on the toxic effects of our urban environments.

Medicine needs the vision of the founder of nursing: our environment is ripe and it is time to clean up the dirty laundry.

Case 41   Dr. Koop: Meet Dr. Ethics

Internet health is going to be big business and there have to be ethics codes. But the transparently corporate codes we have seen so far don't get the job done.

You would never think of getting an annual medical exam over the Internet. Your clinician has to poke and prod you, take your blood, and look you over before your checkup is complete. Some kinds of medicine just don't translate into html.

But if you are visiting your doc about a problem, and you know how to use the Internet, odds are that you will show up with web search results and even detailed studies about your health problems. Your doctor may not like it, but you may know more about the state of research on your condition than he or she does. And because that is true, these days you may join a growing group who skip their checkup and order their drug of choice online from a web drug vendor in Mexico.

Where sensitive issues are concerned, like sex and sexually transmitted diseases, lots of patients would just as soon skip the part where they have to tell Dr. Condemnation about what they did last weekend. For this and many other reasons, Internet health sites are beginning to look like a pretty profitable venture.

The big boys of the Internet health world – WebMD, DrKoop.com, and OnHealth – may not be reporting big corporate earnings yet (one, DrKoop.com, looks like it is well on the way to bankruptcy), but millions of dollars are poured into these sites by advertisers hoping that when you search for web pages about herpes you will find not only medical information but also a clickable link to their company; maybe even a coupon you can use to try to leverage a prescription when you see your doctor.

Blurred boundaries

American physicians have made it perfectly clear that where the Internet and patients are concerned, docs better be cautious about self-educated web-headed patients. "A little [web] information is a dangerous thing," said one prominent editor of a major medical journal. Most physicians know about and have used the Internet in some way, but that doesn't mean that HMOs, hospitals, medical associations or consumer groups have developed good rules for how to guide clinicians whose patients show up with laser-printed medical articles framed by ads for drugs.

The onslaught of direct-to-consumer advertising that has come along with the gold rush in Internet health has everyone confused. It has blurred the boundaries between advertising and journalism, between science and malarkey, and between profiteering and fair business practice. Already all of the major health sites on the Internet have been subject to severe scrutiny for their financial relationships, ranging from simple conflict of interest (can a web site really endorse hospitals who pay a fee?) to complex collusion (when is a medical web site really medical, really corporate, or really free?) and violations of privacy (does your browser cookie from Joe's Internet Health Shop really need to store information about which drug ads you click?). No one has really studied the impact of the Internet on patient care. What has happened though is a rush to write and push "codes of ethics" for Internet healthcare. In response to pressure from patients and physicians alike to enforce codes of conduct for Internet medical sites, three codes of ethics have been produced in the past few years, both sponsored by insiders in the Internet health industry.

The first code was written by the DrKoop.com company, just a couple of months after Koop and his company were flogged in the media for engaging in an egregious conflict of interest by endorsing hospitals who had paid fees to the site. You probably haven't heard much about the other two codes of ethics, each written by a brand new health coalition, because despite the high profile of those who wrote the codes of ethics and their ethicist consultants, neither code applied to anyone who wanted to ignore it.

What we need to help patients and doctors deal with the Internet is a code of ethics for medical web sites. Right? Wrong. Ironically, the most dangerous thing in Internet healthcare may be simple codes of ethics. Why? If the failure of a code of ethics to save DrKoop.com from implosion doesn't convince you, just look at the rest of the Internet, and it becomes clear that systematic, bureaucratic rule-making for the web is dead, dead, dead.

No matter who makes the rules, the Internet has always been a place for individual users to ignore them and create alternative systems of making and distributing information. In the case of healthcare, Internet health sites promise to take a lot of the money out of hospitals, specialist clinical care, and medical publishing by replacing time spent with physicians with time spent on the Internet.

Dozens of little sites in Mexico, Canada, or Poland are selling drugs to anyone who can answer a questionnaire, despite the obvious rules against such conduct out in the great unwired world of medicine. There are some problems with that behavior, ethical and otherwise. But the big boys in Internet health have another big incentive to come up with a code of ethics that shuts out these little players, and fast: money.

Little sites that don't follow rules can grab tons of traffic and make it less profitable to sell ads to big medical companies at the big sites. Not surprisingly, then, both of these new codes of ethics read like a business plan for world domination, calling for every Internet medical site to have an impossibly expensive set of privacy protocols, a huge staff of clinical evaluators, and other bells and whistles no small Internet health site could afford. Neither does a good job defining the important ethical issues that have plagued Dr. Koop and other big players, like the difference between an endorsement, an advertisement and a "sponsored article," or the responsibility of web sites for hazards caused by products they discuss or promote. And the effect of the codes of ethics that have been proposed would be devastating for non-US health sites and for alternative medicine, who could never meet the technical standards.

Internet health is going to be big business and there have to be rules, sanctions and rewards for good practice. But a real code of ethics for health information on the Internet can't be produced until someone actually studies the effect of web sites on health. Once we have data, we need conversation and the little players have to have a voice too.

A code of ethics from the big players is really just a Trojan horse: It looks like a great idea right up until the point where you see that the authors have designed a world in which only two or three medical web sites can survive, and each amounts to little more than a shill for drug advertising. Or perhaps the lesson of Napster is that no matter how hard you try to keep the old business plan together in the Internet world, information has a way of poking its way through, until the leaks collapse the dam.

Case 42   Organ Donation:
Why Isn't There an App for That?

We have come a long way in regard to our attitudes about directed donation for organs since 2005. Back then, Alex Crionas was being refused a direct donation from a willing donor (a friend of his) because, two years prior, Alex had set up a web site, www.SelflessAct.net, to ask for someone to donate to him. Alex says that his friend – the prospective donor – was not recruited through the web site. But it isn't selling, according to the *Tampa Tribune*:

> Because Crionas had set up a web site that was deemed to be in violation of its ethics policy, LifeLink, a Tampa-based organ transplant center, has refused to perform the living donor transplant that Crionas hoped would occur by March. In early February, the center abruptly stopped an evaluation process to determine if 23-year-old Patrick Garrity would be a good match for Crionas.

What isn't clear in the story is why the web site matters if the donor does not come from that venue. The letter to Crionas reads like a disciplinary action from a high school principal:

> His case had been reviewed, the letter said. "In addition, we have reviewed your personal web site." The American Society of Transplant Surgeons and

94

LifeLink are "strongly opposed to the solicitation of organs or organ donors by recipients or their agents through web sites," the letter continued. "After careful deliberation, we will not consider any living donor for you."

If it is in fact the case that the two didn't meet through the web site, it is really, really hard to figure out how a transplant program could arrive at the conclusion that the existence of the web site is enough to exclude any possible directed donor. In fact the decision seems pretty peculiar all the way around because the letter doesn't specify the degree to which the web site played a role in the decision. But on the other hand, this situation does raise the question of how a transplant program can disentangle claims about donor motivations when something like this web site is in evidence . . .

Now fast forward to 2011. Now people waiting on the transplant recipient list put out calls on Facebook and Twitter for organ donors regularly – and they successfully find them. Sarah Taylor, a 53-year-old woman with renal failure for eight years, posted a message on her wall asking for a kidney donor. More than 200 people responded, including her actual donor who was a childhood friend who lived just two blocks away from her. Forty-four-year-old Carlos Sanchez posted a message on Facebook about his need for a kidney transplant. Two minutes later, his town's mayor answered his request. She donated him a kidney and the transplant was successful.

Clearly we've come a long way from when web sites (so 2005) could thwart a potential organ transplant to using social networks to find desperately needed organs. Perhaps the United Network for Organ Sharing is looking a little outdated, or at least should include a social networking component, or maybe an app?

Case 43 Docu-Medical Shows Lack Reality

with Summer Johnson McGee

How can you tell when your nation's healthcare system has collapsed? When television producers attempt to portray our dysfunctional system as great American drama.

The first sign: the creation of a television program that offers access to healthcare to the desperately ill as a prize. "Miracle Workers," formerly appearing on ABC, offered the services of "miracle doctors" to people with horrible medical problems. The show's web site says that the program is an example of the network's "tradition of developing reality programming that makes impossible dreams come true." Access to quality healthcare is now an "impossible dream." Sad, but perhaps true.

And in the grand tradition of ABC medical "docu-dramas," two subsequent shows *Hopkins* and *Boston Med* have also aired, depicting the trials and tribulations of those attempting to access our broken healthcare system.

In a nutshell, these show find people with serious medical problems who nonetheless have the right stuff to be appealing as well as suitably grateful to their television benefactors. The program matches them up with teams of doctors and nurses who have been selected for their buccaneering style, willingness to push the envelope and good looks.

So how exactly does a show that hooks up desperate patients with hospitals falling over one another for the free publicity their best and brightest docs can create square with our healthcare system? Watch the show and you will know that if you are lucky, comb your hair and are willing to dispense with any semblance of privacy, a TV producer and his medical advisers may show up at your house and direct you to a team of well-scrubbed young healthcare professionals with loads of time to spend with you.

These benefactors will smooth the way to your treatment and follow-up care by picking up whatever part of the tab you cannot pay. That is healthcare reality-TV style.

Even worse, it picks the most extreme cases and acts as though this is real medicine. It will make Americans believe that *House* is in fact how every day medicine is practiced. Out of eight hours of TV drama America will see: a double-lung transplant, a face transplant (*American Journal of Bioethics* style), pediatric heart surgery.

What happened to primary care? Oh, I forgot – runny noses and flu shots don't make very good television.

But that is precisely the problem. By glamorizing the highest tech, highest cost, highest drama healthcare in this country, Americans think that this is the most important kind of healthcare, the care to which they are entitled, the care that we all would be lost without.

Bioethicists George Annas and Art Caplan have raised ethical questions for the patients and physicians who actually participate in the shows themselves, but I am much less concerned with whether a patient actually gave their full and free informed consent to be on an hour of prime-time television than the message that this hour of prime-time television conveys to millions of Americans.

House has already given us a sense that every test and every procedure can and ought to be done in American hospitals and these medical "docudramas" will just be just another instrument playing in that same band.

Meanwhile, on the commercial breaks, we are bombarded with ads telling us to buy drugs because a man can throw a football through a tire in his backyard thereby arousing his mate or a butterfly will alight on our pillow if we swallow a capsule when we cannot sleep.

No one has any idea why anything costs what it does whether it be drugs or medical care, but trust us when we tell you it would be dangerous to go to another country to get the same drug at a much lower price. The strategy of the payers hired to look out for our health is to routinely turn down requests for reimbursement in the hopes that we will simply give up.

What is really irritating about shows like *Miracle Workers* is that the show makes healthcare seem a privilege, something you are lucky to get, rather than something you should have as a matter of right. On the flip side, shows like *Hopkins* and *Boston Med* venerate the most expensive, extreme cases in medical care and treat them as though they are routine. It suggests that what is most exciting about medicine occurs on the frontier, as if having your migraines treated, your alcoholism rehabilitated, your back pain relieved, your wheelchair properly sized or your congestive heart failure managed would not be miraculous if they happened today for everyone with these problems.

Worse still, these shows send out the message minute after phony minute that there is hope. Well, if you have a lot of money there is or a television producer in your back pocket. If you don't, then this show is about as close as you are going to get to cutting-edge healthcare.

Note

1. Stat.: A previous version of this story incorrectly said that 45 to 100 million Americans die each year of medical mistakes.

Caution **Eight**

You Aren't Dead Until Someone Tells You So

Case 44   Redefining Retirement: Beyond Rest and Recreation

I want to live a long, long time. Walks in the forest and on the beach convince me of my love for life, and my heart skips a beat at the sight and smell of a baby. When I see an old friend or swim in a cool pond or ski down a steep hill, when I see the sun rise, I know I am alive. What I am not so sure about is living a long time in a world where there isn't much to do or where the opportunities to flourish are few and ill-defined.

Retirement planning is a product of a world where people did not live much longer than the expected retirement age. With a gold watch, the parents of today's retirees went home, or to warmer climates, at age 60 or so, to spend a few years covered by the security of a social net that was designed to keep them comfortable for precisely that amount of time.

But then one has to consider the changing world of medicine, which is conducting an all-out attack on the diseases and conditions that define aging today. Improvements in public health and the environment are attacking aging from another front. But either way I could live much, much longer than did my grandparents. And I want to live, to feel that breeze, smell that season, surge, with the energy of youth.

But that is the rub. The love for the vigor of life that drives so many Americans to retire at 50 or 60 into a life of "leisure" is not matched by a world that accommodates those who tune out of the work world.

Bioethics for Beginners: 60 Cases and Cautions from the Moral Frontier of Healthcare,
First Edition. Glenn McGee.
© 2012 John Wiley & Sons, Ltd. Published 2012 by John Wiley & Sons, Ltd.

The institutions of the western world, from employers to religions to government to insurance and hospitals, are all set up as though life after 60 is a downhill slide, free from responsibility and devoid of heroes.

Unless there is another great recession, my retirement plan will allow me to retire in my 60s too. But if I am as healthy as the average 60-year-old in the United States, I might have 30 or even 40 years more to live.

But in America it is hard to get old, and it will get harder, because while we may be able to extend youthful powers into the mid-100s, those who have those powers will not have the opportunities that define growth and vigor.

If we are going to build a world that supports early retirement and nearly eternal life, we better get busy making sure that it isn't a boring world. Nursing homes, casinos and shopping malls are already filled nearly to capacity with those bored out of their minds by a world that has no use for the minds and hearts of the aging – only for their wallets.

It is time to redefine retirement, which will no longer be rest for the weary or a perpetual vacation. Retirement should be viewed as a special time for those with lots of wisdom, experience, and accumulated skills to play new and important roles in society.

Case 45   Medicare Is Going South: What Do We Owe the Aging?

It doesn't take a crystal ball to see that the Medicare population will soon double as baby boomers hit 65. And even a cynic can't miss the daily news about what's brewing in biotechnology: treatments for just about everything that kills us.

Stem cells, gene therapy, new surgeries, and better drugs are coming. Imagine the baby boomers still going strong in the year 2015: Alzheimer's and Parkinson's diseases may be cured, most heart diseases will be treatable, and tumors will mostly get stopped in their tracks.

This great news for boomers may be big trouble for the economy. The research and treatments that will provide new organs and better lifestyles for the aging will cost a fortune. The present Medicare system cannot pay for the new medicine on the horizon.

The fight to stabilize Medicare is more important than most legislators understand, even after the passage of the Affordable Care Act. Everyone agrees that Americans should ensure that our aging have decent care but how we define the standard of decent is entirely another question. It is a long-standing American ethic that everyone must pitch in to provide a good life for our elders – but not too good of a life, not one that will bankrupt the current working generation in the process.

Think big

Social security too is on the ropes already, with most contributions from those in their 30s and 40s going directly to those already on the rolls. Even the best organized AARP lobbying effort cannot hide the fact that we are going to have to make some tough choices.

We have to think bigger than Medicare. We have to change the way we think about getting old. Retirement at 65 is an artifact of an era when work meant back-breaking labor.

Tomorrow's jobs don't have to be so stressful that only the young can participate. The American dream of retirees running away to a beach house is going to have to go south for most Americans.

Aging Americans need to stay in the work force, so that the talents and wisdom of our elders is not lost. And there is no reason to expect the nation to subsidize 30 or 40 years of leisure time for capable and experienced workers.

Retirement is a nice idea that has had devastating consequences: when the aging leave American cities for suburbs and retirement communities, our cities decay and the burden of paying for schools and hospitals falls entirely on the same urban middle class that subsidizes Medicare.

The Medicare debate is about social justice and medical ethics. Americans agree that we must care for the aging. But Medicare makes some pretty weird assumptions about what it means to age.

It is time to think ahead about how we are going to pay for the amazing discoveries that will lengthen and improve our lives. The aging want to live meaningful, not just healthy, lives. We owe it to them and to our community to rethink what we want aging to mean. Retirement is an idea that has outlived its usefulness.

Case 46   The Fight to Die Well: We Will Expect More from Death Than Our Ancestors Did

We die hard, working to cheat the grim reaper every step of the way. If any civilization in history loved to live, our own would surely rank among them. Obviously, twenty-first-century western society lives with gusto, fighting each battle and building each bridge with the élan of a bloated prizefighter. The twenty-first century is a testimony to nothing so much as the will of western societies to fight against their own dying.

Take a look at our technologies: seat belts and safe cars, environmental protection, child safety and labor laws, weather forecasting. We fight to die well, too. Twentieth-century Americans set up life insurance, invented Medicare and Social Security, and made up a new kind of tool called the "advance directive" to give the dying more power over how they die. In the twenty-first century (what we have experienced of it so far), we have mandated health insurance for even those with pre-existing conditions, allowed for Medicare to reimburse for time spent helping our elders complete their advance directive and even have embraced palliative care.

Never letting go

Truly, ours is a generation that has struggled to strike a balance between the eastern tradition of venerating ancestors and the western tendency to, well, get them out of the way of progress.

We also refuse to let anything about us die. I'm not talking about the odd new habit of freezing heads, bodies, or other parts in liquid nitrogen so that one day we can awaken, like Woody Allen's *Sleeper*, to live forever in the world of *The Jetsons*. No, I'm talking about metaphorical death.

We don't like the idea of losing our identity, and we are the first civilization to make ideas "permanent." The library burned at Alexandria and the work of millions was lost. The first films from the first part of this century are gone. But these words you are reading, however paltry, have the potential to live on forever, protected in perpetuity by the astonishingly resilient thing called computing. It is a central theme of our time that books may get remaindered, but e-mail and web pages could well live forever. Everyone from Timothy Leary to Darth Vader lives on in the Internet.

Dying well

Our death rites will change. There just isn't enough real estate to bury the American dead. There aren't enough transplant organs. And it isn't sufficient for most folks to write a simple will.

The twenty-first century will not see the death of death. People will still grow old, and they will still die. But the clues for how death will change are already present. We will live longer and better as we age. We will age more gracefully. We will expect more from death than did our ancestors, and expect more, too, from our children and grandchildren and great-grand-children. The recent trend of late divorce – divorce after age 70 – suggests that people expect more from their own relationships as they get older. When we do finally die in the twenty-first century, our death rites will change. There just isn't enough real estate to bury the American dead. There aren't enough transplant organs. And it isn't sufficient for most folks to write a simple will. After all, we can use the cells, sperm, and eggs of the dead these days for reproductive purposes, and we can even go back and figure out who Thomas Jefferson slept with. The dead don't rest easy anymore. So dying will increasingly mean planning ahead.

Nobody likes to think about dying, and death in the next century will not be any easier to grasp. But coping with death, coming to die, and passing over into death are all going to be a little better as we develop policies, rules, ethics, and technologies that make bioethics a part of a twenty-first century death. Even if we can't cheat the reaper.

Case 47   The Case of the Body Snatchers

When it comes to the body, they say you can't take it with you when you die. But they didn't say it should be sold from the back of a truck. Or that you should not have the right to give a fully informed consent for whatever it is that medical science wants to do with your remains.

Criminals have been stealing bones from bodies at crematoriums in New York and New Jersey. They were then sold to for-profit tissue banks in New Jersey and Florida. Among the victims was the late host of PBS television's Masterpiece Theater, British broadcaster and journalist Alistair Cooke. His bones were removed without his or his family's permission or even knowledge, and then sold for thousands of dollars. What happened to Cooke has happened to others.

Investigations across the United States have revealed a gruesome market in body parts made possible by a motley collection of grim reapers who sometimes secretly and illegally and with dubious consent harvest the skin, bones, tendons, organs, and even brains of those in funeral homes, burial sites and morgues. From Maine to California to Louisiana, un-scrupulous brokers are removing tissues and selling them to tissue banks that then sell them to medical schools, hospitals, research institutes, and testing facilities. The trade in tissues is a half-billion dollar industry and that is enough to get some who have access to body parts to put their ethics on the shelf.

There is a long and ignoble history of pseudo-medical mutilation of bodies: William Burke and William Hare in the nineteenth century murdered and robbed graves to supply bodies for examination to the school of medicine in Edinburgh. A pathologist present at the Princeton, N.J., hospital where Albert Einstein died, removed Einstein's eyes and his brain, despite his specific instructions that he be cremated. The brain went off to Philadelphia, was divided into dozens of slices and preserved; it then spent the next 40 years being lugged around the United States by various doctors and speculators. A friend of Elvis' barber in Memphis promises to make a clone of the King from his stash of slick black hair that he kept without Presley's knowledge. A San Francisco museum came under attack for its exhibit of the filleted bodies of what some said were Chinese prisoners who had been executed and who obviously had no chance to consent to their remains being put on display. Tulane University in Louisiana has admitted that it sold seven cadavers to a distributor who resold them for a sizable profit to the US Army for use in land-mine testing. There is record demand for organs and tissues from the dead. Every year hundreds of thousands of tissue transplants are done. Most of these tissues are given in response to legitimate requests for their use from reputable organizations such as eye and skin banks. But, unlike organ procurement, which has strict oversight from the federal government, tissue procurement does not. And there are sleazy operators out there among the many good guys ready to remove a bone from grandpa's leg at the funeral home or remove an entire brain at the morgue to send to a research institute without the fully informed consent of the donor or the family.

Research firms, pharmaceutical companies, government agencies, and even the military have uses for almost every body part you can name. We now know how to use the dead to help the living. The public policy problem is that there is enough money changing hands that some who deal with the dead are dispensing with consent and yanking parts out of people who have given no indication that they wanted to be donors.

Tissue banks bring in hundreds of millions of dollars in the legal sale of parts from the deceased who have agreed that their bodies can be used as sources of bone and ligament which can be sterilized, shaped, and transplanted into others. But existing regulations and oversight are not enough. With so many people competing for the bodies of so few, and with lax laws governing the trade of tissues from the dead, it was inevitable that some who seem to have learned their dissection skills from watching *The Sopranos* would enter the business.

It is one thing to fear death, but another to fear the desecration of a family member. Organ donation and much of the most important biomedical research depends on the generosity of donors, and that in turn depends on trust. The public will not support organ and tissue donation if Americans are worried that someone is getting away with stealing the parts of their loved ones. And that would be a tragedy since organ and tissue donation save lives. It is time for the federal government to wake up and get involved in regulating the tissue trade before mistreating the dead starts to cost lives.

Case 48   A Few Conclusions from the Terri Schiavo Case

Living wills may not work, but I'm getting one

There couldn't be a more salient test of the question as to what it might mean if I do not write down "I prefer not to be held hostage by fears about a feeding tube for more than a decade, please." I've argued in several papers that living wills are a mistake and are unlikely to work, and others have found enough empirical evidence to cast doubt on the idea that advance directives make much difference in the care that patients receive. But tell that to Michael Schiavo. Today it is awfully clear that no matter what I and other critics of living wills might have believed about how well they work, they do at least make it easier to avoid the Schiavo level of confusion and wrangling. I have opined over and over again that living wills are too litigious.

Um, ok, I was wrong. All around the country people will now begin thinking very seriously about writing down their wishes about feeding tubes and respirators. It is as John Danforth said when he pushed for the Patient Self-Determination Act in the first place: young people "should get a *Miranda* warning" about what can happen if they do not talk to others about healthcare preferences.

An advance directive aimed at ensuring that your doctors and significant others know what treatments you would, or would not, want has suddenly become the most important tool one could have in the event that there is any difference between your views and your family's views about end of life care. Country simple: if you would want a feeding tube removed were you in persistent vegetative state, and you think that it is enough that you told your family as much, think again and get a living will. Warning: not guaranteed to protect you against the combined legislative force of a majority of Congress.

In the future, it will be tough to get a majority of legislators
to agree to support choices by individuals about healthcare

The scene on the House floor as the debate persisted about Schiavo was staggering. Those who fought for the sanctity of marriage now fight against the importance of a husband's choice. Those who fought for the importance of the tenth amendment and states' rights more generally are suddenly desperately fighting against a state's rule of law. The body that made it possible for *Cruzan*'s case to become the Patient Self Determination Act is now deciding that expressed views about dying just don't matter. Why? Because Democrats do not want to run for office against campaign commercials that feature Terri Schiavo dying.

The fallout from this case will be that legislators will not want to interfere with decisions about life and death for fear that they will be pegged as insufficiently caring about human life, or worse a rationer. This is precisely what we saw in the ridiculous debate over "Death Panels" in the summer of 2009.

Quality end of life care is now officially less important than Jack
Kevorkian and Terri Schiavo

The battle over Terri Schiavo is illuminated by a single, vulnerable woman. Nothing works better as a political motivator than a simple poster child. If Democrats could have managed to make a symbol out of a young woman dying of a curable chronic disease because she has no insurance, we might have had healthcare reform all that much sooner. And the lesson doesn't end there: the Schiavo case sucked the life out of the end of life care debate. Just as Kevorkian turned the nation's attention away from the problems that made his services seem desirable, the Schiavo case turned our attention away from dozens of critical questions about the funding of hospice, palliative care, and a dozen other issues related to how we treat people at the end of life.

People struggle most against the worst odds

There is no question about Terri Schiavo's condition. She is never ever going to awaken, no, to be more blunt, her brain is utterly destroyed and there is nothing of what was Terri Schiavo remaining in her but the simple functioning stem that causes her other organs to continue to function at the most basic level. That much is clear. All that remains of Terri Schiavo is her dignity and the symbolic meaning of her body. So why does anyone fight to keep her in this condition rather than discontinuing a treatment that everyone agrees is not therapeutic? What does it mean to fight against the impossible in this case? Republicans fighting against this measure have tried desperately to avoid discussion of what might re-grow Ms. Schiavo's brain, because God forbid they say what the man who offered Mr. Schiavo $1 million to keep Terri Schiavo said: stem cells.[1] No, there is nothing here for them to point to but miracle. And it should be noted that pushing for a miracle against impossible scientific odds is a critical part of the American culture in an era in which physicians often feel that they must offer treatments that they do not believe are therapeutic. The idea that patients and others have a right to request things whether or not they work is being reinforced right now.

Compassion for the dying Schiavo and her family ought not be lost

There was no question in my mind that the Schiavo case illustrates wanton, callous political maneuvering on the part of some. It was equally clear to me that Congress has no business working on this case in this way – interfering in the lives of those who are touched by such tragedy as they make private decisions. But it should not be lost that many who have begun to fight in this matter as it has been quickly escalated have deep compassion for the Schiavos, and that such compassion came from a vital sense that death and suffering must be understood and respected – and that love for life is important and beautiful. Somewhere in the middle is the opportunity to take this case and use it to move quickly to reform of national policies for end of life care. I hope that happens.

Case 49   Living Wills Save Money? Dude, Did You Really Say That Out Loud?

Having an advance directive explicating your wishes for end-of-life care just makes sense right? Well apparently some are arguing that it makes "cents" as well.

Former HHS Secretary Mike Leavitt made the incredible blunder of claiming that living wills for senior citizens could "reduce Medicare's skyrocketing healthcare costs." Why? Duh, he replied, because the old people will die faster. The actual reasons for Leavitt's conclusions were left vague. Leavitt proposed, years prior to the ACA, that physicians who bill Medicare must include a discussion of the directives in their consultations with patients. And nobody disputes that such a discussion is a good idea, or even that it might "work" in terms of getting patients' wishes on the table. But the question of whether living wills actually change outcomes in hospitals is still very much alive. There is data, but it isn't conclusive. More to the point, whether or not living wills save money would depend entirely on what people actually say in their living wills – and nothing will scare aging folks more than the idea that the government wants them to sign living wills because that way they'll die less expensively. Even if it were true – which it very likely is not – it speaks volumes about how difficult it has been to discuss advance directives in public policy without pushing hot buttons.

However, after the passage of ACA, it is clear that physicians can and will reimburse for having "the conversation" with Medicare patients. Advance directive discussion will even have a billing code. So now do you believe that advance directives will save money, at least for Medicare? I hate to be cynical (but I am) and it is clear that the medicalization of and billing for advance care planning could only have been justified (even if only behind closed doors) by enormous savings for Medicare.

But then, is that really a bad thing? Our elderly will be able to express their wishes to their physicians and loved ones and the government will save a few (trillion) pennies. Seems like a win-win to me.

Case 50   The Plural of Anecdote Is Not Ambien

The media has no idea how to deal with case reports.

A few years ago Princeton health economist Uwe Reinhardt, Dartmouth geriatrician Joann Lynn, and I filmed a documentary on the effect of advancing biomedical technology on affordable healthcare in the United States. Five hours of interviews were reduced to 10-minute bookends for a set of short, emotional stories that obliterated the complexities of the issues. As Reinhardt quipped in our cab, repeating the oft-cited quote, the plural of anecdote is not data. Except on television.

We've all had this experience: You bring work home and talk about concepts central to biomedical research such as evidence-based medicine, controlled trials, equipoise, peer-review, or impact factor. Friends' eyes roll up into their skulls in boredom. Yet the same topics come up in everyday conversation all the time, just framed in a different way: "I know a person who lost his house to the cost of drugs," and "you know a guy who is alive because of Lipitor." Heated arguments ensue about real problems in science, but driven by someone's single story.

Stories are not the enemy of good science and evidence-based medicine. Physicians make crucial but subtle changes in their practices based on individual experiences. Scientists all use intuition and inductive reasoning in the nascent period of an investigation. But anecdotes cannot substitute for either ethnography or controlled study. When Terri Schiavo became the world's test case for diagnosing persistent vegetative state (PVS), the emotional intonations about Ms. Schiavo waking up began to sound like Intelligent Design.

A paradox of biomedical research is that huge controlled trials, meta-analyses, and reviews of the literature are ubiquitous, but the number of "case reports" – and journals comprised entirely of incidental "findings" – is growing.

The media has no idea how to deal with case reports. The worst example of this in recent times was a case study of Zolpidem, the nonbenzodiazepine-branded "Ambien" and approved by the US Food & Drug Administration for the treatment of insomnia. Physicians Ralf Clauss and Wally Nel have published, a few cases at a time, their very different use of the medication. The Guardian carried a breathless report of Clauss et al.'s August report in the journal *NeuroRehabilitation* of three cases involving patients who have been in PVS, they report, for more than three years.[2] Claus and Nel grabbed the front page with the *Guardian*'s report that they used Ambien to wake up these patients.

The "investigators" had administered Zolpidem for between three and six years and saw each of the three "treated" patients wake up each day as a result of the medication; one even "caught a baseball." When the medication wore off, the patients dropped back into PVS each evening.

Stunning science? It seemed so, too, back in 2000, when Claus and a different set of South African colleagues published in the *South African Medical Journal* on a single case with essentially the same outcome. In 2001 they made the same claim in a letter to the same journal. At no point did the investigators conduct an actual study of the phenomenon, with an IRB-approved research protocol or informed consent. Again and again they "wrote up" their "cases," describing their work as innovative medical management rather than research. Journal editors, asleep at the switch, have been derelict in publishing bad research disguised as cases – in this instance a case with the impact of finding a life-extending potion or the presence of extraterrestrial life.

Investigators who jumpstart their programs with case reports are often in search of research support, as was Claus – who as a result of the case report is now funded. In this respect they, and the journals who publish nothing but these case reports, are like the television producers I worked with: They aim at using the power of stories to make the claims and reap the rewards that come from research, but without doing the research. The victims are journalists, readers, and in the *Claus* case the patients and their families, who are exposed to uncontrolled experiments framed as good medicine. It is time for editors, journalists, the FDA, and the US Health & Human Services Office for Human Research Protections (OHRP) to clamp down on the "case study."

Notes and References

1. CNN/Reuters reported that a California businessman offered Michael Schiavo, husband of Terri Schiavo, $1 million, "to relinquish his custodial rights to Terri's parents in an effort to keep the hope for Terri alive," Herring told a Los Angeles news conference. "After viewing video of Terri on television, I came to the belief that there was hope for her . . . I have seen miraculous recoveries occur through the use of stem cells in patients suffering a variety of conditions," Herring said.
2. S. Boggan, "Reborn," *Guardian*, September 12, 2006. Accessed at: www. guardian.co.uk/science/2006/sep/12/health.healthandwellbeing.

Caution **Nine**

Eat Only Food for Thought

Case 51   Fat in America

It is always diet season in America, always time to squeeze into a dress or swimsuit. Americans are more overweight than any people of the world, and infinitely more obsessed about it. Ads for liposuction clinics keep local magazines afloat. And everyone knows someone who takes a diet drug, or who took fen-phen, or who abuses diet, herbs, exercise, or laxatives in pursuit of a better body.

Men too are dieting in record numbers to meet an ever-more-fit male standard for health. And recent studies reveal that even young American children experience the throes of anorexia and bulimia, and more and more parents worry early about the fat baby.

Discrimination against the obese has been documented so many times that litigation for it has become commonplace.

We spend more than $10 billion annually on dieting, which fails to accomplish long-term results more than 99 percent of the time. Imagine a society that spends 300 times more on weight loss than on prenatal care, 1,000 times more on weight loss than on housing the homeless, and 6,000 times more on it than on physical education in our public schools.

How we see our expanding waistline says a lot about us as a society. Being fat is expensive – food costs money, sedentary behavior is inefficient and reports continually document the long-term health risks of obesity. We could debate the fact that society as a whole supports the health cost of any of our risky behaviors – driving too fast, drinking alcohol, living on hurricane-swept coastline. But who among us would pass a sin test for health insurance?

Bioethics for Beginners: 60 Cases and Cautions from the Moral Frontier of Healthcare, First Edition. Glenn McGee.
© 2012 John Wiley & Sons, Ltd. Published 2012 by John Wiley & Sons, Ltd.

Virtual living

We are a people that explore, a people that welcome struggle, a people that think on our feet. We are the society that mastered technology and converted it into products and powers.

But, as David Shenk chronicles in his exceptional book, *The End of Patience: More Notes of Caution on the Information Revolution*, the technologies that seem to liberate us can create their own prison. Our lives are lived through virtual-this and artificial-that. We don't go west to surf anymore. We do it from the sofa in Jersey. Most Americans get their exercise riding a stationary bicycle – a bike ride that never goes anywhere.

Philosopher William James said human beings need the "moral equivalent of war." When we are at peace, we rot. James said we need a struggle against an enemy and an urgent goal to keep us alive. His words inspired FDR to create the CCC, an agency that built much of the nation's new infrastructure of dams and bridges by putting Americans to work. His words inspired John F. Kennedy, who mentioned them in creating the Peace Corps. It is time for the moral equivalent of war. We are a people whose disease is not our obesity, but our lack of inspiration.

Geek heroes

Ours is a generation of geek heroes, men and women who changed the world by inventing plastic boxes that think for us. The web you're surfing is the world we have created in their image. We want to live in that world but with the body of Mr. Atlas, the guy who kicks sand on Bill Gates at the beach.

Get real. Weight loss is a stupid goal for virtually all of the American population. Weight loss has to be a byproduct of a change in the way we see life and living. It is time to put some of our diet money into innovative new ways to flourish that use our bodies and our minds. Our nation needs a new volunteer effort, to clean up the streets and build houses and fight fires and teach little kids to play soccer. The answer is surprisingly simple: advertising. Here's the ad: LOSE 10 POUNDS NOW WITH UNIQUE HAMMER AND NAIL METHOD. The weight we lose might just be the chip on our shoulder.

Case 52 Breakfast for Thought

You've probably heard by now about the latest trend from across the Atlantic: fear of food. It has become a recreational activity all over Europe to protest genetically modified food and crops. Doesn't sound like fun to you?

You just haven't gotten scared yet. As an American dolt, lulled by the convenience of the modern world, you probably love the great taste, skillful preparation, and neat experience of American food and foods from new cultures and cuisine.

Just another American victim of corporate greed, you like shopping for new kinds of food, prepared in advance or in nifty packages. Silly Americans.

You will catch on soon, because the rhetoric is heating up. In the first six months of 1999 alone, 170 magazine pieces and more than 1,000 newspaper articles joined the debate about so called GM foods, made with genetic engineering. That number has surely grown ten-fold in the intervening years. The accusation is simple: things that are engineered are hazardous to your health, and you better not eat them or you will keel over dead, and quick.

Americans are slow to challenge technology. We know all about engineering and we like it. Small farmers, beer makers, village grocers, and florists, to name a few American icons, owe their careers to food engineering and have been mixing plants with other plants for a very long time.

Indeed, genetic engineering of food stuff source crops is at least as old as civilization, beginning with the very first attempts to cultivate crops in Africa and the Mideast.

Wacky food is also very American. Europeans might not mind having one or two flavors of breakfast cereal, but we have been choosing among hundreds of flake-and-nut-and-marshmallow-bit concoctions to eat with our Tang for almost a century. Powders, microwaves and lemon-lime-oranges are all the stuff of what we frequently praise as American ingenuity.

Where Europeans have often preferred a pastoral concept of food, opting for grainy toast and marmalade instead of frosted Pop Tarts, we tend to think of food as a product, as part of a lifestyle of convenience and as the cornerstone of an enormous American agricultural and chemical economy.

But the new genetic engineering, we are being told by our European friends, is different and bad. Foes of GM foods point to weird combinations: lobster genes in lettuce, insect genes in tomatoes.

They identify some scary potential health risks: a gene in a genetically modified pig causes problems when you eat bacon, or a large quantity of

112

genetically modified fruit causes a cancerous change in human cells. These are pretty scary possibilities.

But it is not yet clear that they are real risks, or risks that compare with, say, the risk associated with drinking bad tap water and diet soda or eating too much of any kind of food, natural or not.

The debate about GM foods is so far just a vote on your feelings about food and engineering. So before you clear out your kitchen cabinets, remember that there is a lot of real research to be done.

The ethical questions are going to be complicated too: Where should we put our energy, into making more natural food or feeding more people in more ways? What kind of rules should govern, for example, kosher GM foods and new nutraceutical foods that carry pharmaceutical properties?

Where GM foods are concerned, there is a lot on our plate.

Case 53 Want Fish? Ethics First, Please

The threat of the ocean's imminent collapse is a new kind of issue for bioethics.

"Eat first, then ethics," wrote German poet Bertolt Brecht. But even Brecht would be horrified by the "fish apocalypse" of 2048 that Boris Worm of Dalhousie University predicts in the November 3, 2006 issue of *Science*. As far as fish are concerned, we appear to be eating not only first, but without forethought, and we never get around to the ethics.

The problem of diminishing saltwater fish populations is not a new one; the United Nations has reported consistently since the mid-1990s that all 17 of the world's major fishing areas have been fished to the point that sustainability is seriously in question for many if not most of the commercially harvested species there. The most famous fishing areas of North American lore, such as the Grand Banks and Georges Bank, have been closed and reopened with hardly any planning, as environmentalist and commercial political lobbies each win their way for a month, year, or decade, but never in a process that ends in stewardship of the oceans.

Those at the top of the fish business' food chain aren't doing so well financially, despite the appearance that industry prevails in matters of regulation of fishing. Both large commercial fisheries and small immigrant families with one boat in places like New Bedford, Mass., find themselves unable to eke out a living from tuna and swordfish and scallops. Fishing doesn't really make much money even for those who have become adept at vacuuming fish from the sea. In response, governments provide subsidies.

That's not enough, however, to sustain fleets and shareholders, so companies turn from fishing cod and the like to fishing the sort of creatures that emerge from the sea so unpalatable that one knows immediately that they will have to be, as Wendell Berry put it, "prettified" until they no longer "resemble anything that ever lived."[1]

Either way, as stocks of fish that were once commercially undesirable have plummeted, large fish, marine mammals, and even birds have been robbed of a big piece of their food chain. And that means we too are affected, as some of our most intimate ecosystems – those that protect and nourish our food and water supply – become, in collapsing, a toxic abyss. Fish species that live near coastlines, reducing the risk of red tide and providing detoxification to water supplies, are disappearing.

The threat of the ocean's imminent collapse is a new kind of issue for bioethics, which you might call "disaster ethics." The problem is that the public is simply uninterested in the catastrophic consequences of decimating fish stocks. Or at least they are until an oil rig explodes in the Gulf of Mexico. Then gulf shrimp and scallops are right out. But until then, and even not so shortly thereafter, debates about ozone holes, stem cells, and the intelligence of the design of life simply pale in comparison to what is likely to happen to our oceans.

The most visible evidence of the "fish problem" is still invisible by comparison to Korean research fraud and votes on healthcare reform. But the fish story is more important by a long shot and requires actions far more simple than choosing a Senator: Stop eating creatures that are being fished to extinction, and tell your friends to stop, too.

Our species may not have crawled out of the oceans to build civilization, but our willingness to protect the oceans is a bulwark not just of the ethics of environmental stewardship but also of the responsibility to keep cities from being poisoned or falling into the ocean and millions from starving to death. It's a pretty high price to pay for sushi.

There's no time to do long-term studies of whether fish are disappearing. We can't eat before our ethics. The ethical decisions the human population makes in this decade about fishing will set into motion a way of thinking and acting about the earth and its ecosystems that will take ethics off the plate entirely for our grandchildren. They will live in a world where the decisions about fish and the oceans have less to do with whether to eat swordfish than about what kind of engineered fish cell they'd like with their chips. Our policy about fishing isn't just fishy; it's bad science coupled with bad ethics. And at the end of the day, that will mean empty nets.

Case 54   Dying for Food

Theresa Schiavo spent more than a decade fighting an eating disorder. As millions recoil in horror at the fact that she died from the removal of a feeding tube, the irony that a woman who was plagued by food should die in that way has been lost. Ms. Schiavo entered her persistent vegetative state, in all likelihood, as a result of a heart attack brought on by her struggle with weight.

But when beautiful people, dressed in clothes too tiny to fit most Americans, host one program after another in which Terri Schiavo is fashioned as a vulnerable symbol of death by starvation, it is all too easy to miss the fact that Terri Schiavo did her "starving" twenty years ago.

Ms. Schiavo made no secret of the fact that she wanted to weigh 85 pounds. Ironically, the photos of her as a svelte, tanned young woman, paraded as pictures of "Terri as a healthy woman" – or as "Terri as she might be again" – were taken in the throes of her battle with food and with bulimia. The pictures and the association with dying "from lack of food" should be familiar to anyone who is familiar with eating disorders. At least seven million Americans suffer from eating disorders like anorexia and bulimia, and 61 percent of cases last a decade or more.

If you are wondering whether or not the Terry Schiavo who had a heart attack would have said that she would want to forego nutrition and hydration, you don't know bulimia. She had already undergone a decade of refusing food at a basic, fundamental level, in the most resolute way imaginable.

At the time that Terri Schiavo went into persistent vegetative state, she had undergone some treatment for her eating disorder, but not much. Today, treatment for bulimia is even more expensive, and the images that torture young women about weight are more obvious and ubiquitous. Terri Schiavo's heart attack was, ultimately, a result of the lack of resources for the treatment of several of the known side effects of eating disorders. There was a lack of support, a lack of comprehensive health-care, and a lack of awareness. What society was ready to offer her is food, and images of "thin." And indeed, that is all anyone outside her hospice offered her at the end of her life: food, pictures of vitality, and an entreaty to endure.

It would have cost society a fortune to do more for the young Ms. Schiavo – and millions like her – than to offer up the paradoxes of American weight consciousness. Treating eating disorders costs a fortune – tens of thousands of dollars a month on average for intensive treatment. Many, many women in particular receive no treatment, and many more are treated too little or for too short a time. Terri Schiavo was not alone in her struggle – but her struggle was not the one embraced by those who venerated life at all costs.

There are dozens of issues about Schiavo that will linger in bioethics for decades, and most of them are much more important, I suppose, than the role of eating disorders in medical and end of life decisions. It is incredibly troubling that patients linger in a vegetative state for decades while we try to figure out how to work together to match the goals of medicine to the importance of compassion. Ultimately, we all seem to know now that it is going to be hard to find a way for even like-minded communities to agree on how to balance life and liberty under circumstances like those of Terri Schiavo.

But it ought to be possible to get the hundreds of millions of Americans who have been watching the battle over Terry Schiavo and food to agree on one thing: people should not be allowed to linger for years in a fully-conscious, suffering-riddled persistent state of self-starvation. More than half the nation struggles with weight, and we are fatter than at any time in our history. And simultaneously, Americans worship beauty in unforgiving ways that provoke as much masochism about weight gain and weight loss as one could imagine.

It is no surprise that Terri Schiavo died when her nutrition and hydration were discontinued. But it should come as a shock that those who fight over nutrition at the end of life are so tolerant of a paternalism about weight and food – an attitude that killed Terri in the first place.

Note and Reference

1. W. Berry, *The Art of the Common-Place: The Agrarian Essays of Wendell Berry* (Washington, D.C: Counterpoint Press, 2002).

Caution Ten

Beware of Ideologues and Demagogues

Case 55 Bioethics for Christians, Corporate Whores, and Atheists

President of the Center for Policy in Emerging Technologies and ultra-conservative bioethicist Nigel Cameron is less than pleased with the role that Christian scholars play in bioethics today.

He says Christians don't get much attention in bioethics anymore. It is hard to disagree with the claim he makes that the dominant views in evidence in bioethics these days are secular. Most bioethics-oriented publications, and those with the most impact in the scientific and medical professions, are undeniably written within the "secular" discourse of bioethics – that is, are written without drawing in a significant way upon theology, or relying on justifications based on God or a Judeo-Christian faith tradition in particular.

Theology and religion both played defining roles in bioethics' origins. "Early" bioethics of the 1970s focused on the "big picture" of environmental and health issues – and there was less focus on esoterica. Theological bioethicists engaged in dialog about big questions like whether or not technology is moving faster than medicine in general, and developed a rich literature about "playing God," to name just two examples. Religious bioethics brought hospital ethics committees into existence. Theologian ethicists and in particular (in the United States) scholars of Christian and of Jewish ethics framed bioethics for close to a decade and used it to shape a new and vigorous debate about ethics in society and ethics in technology.

Bioethics for Beginners: 60 Cases and Cautions from the Moral Frontier of Healthcare,
First Edition. Glenn McGee.
© 2012 John Wiley & Sons, Ltd. Published 2012 by John Wiley & Sons, Ltd.

What happened to religious bioethics?

Well, according to Cameron, Arthur Caplan, arguably one of America's two or three best known public intellectuals, and director of the University of Pennsylvania Center for Bioethics, happened. Cameron writes:

> Arthur Caplan is the quintessential face of contemporary bioethics. Yet he does not in any way represent the American people. How did bioethics get so out of whack with the people? How did it switch from a Hippocratic focus on the sanctity of life to a public relations department for whatever the biotech industry wants to do next? ... [The] central problem, of course, is that we walked out. There is no question that a chief agent of secularization in American culture has been "conservative" Christians.[1]

Tough love from Nigel: "Caplan is a charming ... the enemy of their enemy is their friend ... guy whose affable manner made the media fall in love with secular bioethics – so Caplan inadvertently opened the doors to the Devil Himself, and behind Caplan is some "wannabe" named Glenn McGee, who is waiting to finish off God and Christian bioethics in particular." That would be me.

The problem with Dr. Cameron's argument isn't that he's wrong on the sociology: the best accounts of the changes in bioethics, identified in particular in books by Tina Stevens, Al Jonsen, and Jennifer K. Walker, really do show that there was a kind of withdrawal by theology scholars from bioethics, just as bioethics would eventually "move out" in large part from philosophy departments. No question either that bioethics has begun to look "secular" in the sense that most bioethics scholars, like most Americans, do not hold Cameron's view that embryonic stem cell research is murder destroys human life, that Terri Schiavo should have been kept alive indefinitely, and that human nature is an essential, unchanging thing given by God to be preserved unaltered by human stewards.

But what is really troubling about his argument is that, like Carl Elliot, Cameron claims that secular bioethics is inherently instrumentalist and at the utter disposal of pharmaceutical companies and biotechnology. Like Elliot he presents no substantial evidence of this, and like Elliot his is a claim that turns the goal of Caplan and others of interacting with the public into a sign of (secular) evangelism on behalf of big Pharma.

It is troubling because it is incredibly hypocritical. There is superficial irony in Cameron's clever but incredibly unscholarly bashing "the likes of Caplan" because he and his wannabes aren't "profound Christian thinkers" like Paul Ramsey. Here is Dr. Cameron, after all, writing in

118

some "insiders" web site on behalf of "moral seriousness" and careful theology. It's not credible. Nigel Cameron, on behalf of pro-life bioethics scholars in his sway, isn't complaining that the serious theologians have left the bioethics building. He isn't complaining that there isn't enough attention to questions about religion in bioethics. He's complaining that the right-to-life movement doesn't have an effective Washington think-tank yet, that it doesn't get enough television time, and that it isn't taken seriously because it uses abortion language and gets labeled as the "religious right." If you don't believe me, check out Cameron's web page, which points to his own serious and scholarly engagement with Nightline, Frontline, CNN, and the BBC. Nothing wrong with that, obviously, but it does rather put a kink in the whole "naughty secularists chase television" argument.

We do need more energy in theological bioethics. More religion departments hiring PhD trained bioethics scholars with theology backgrounds. More bioethics centers seeking out, hiring and promoting theologians in their midst. More representation of theologians in bioethics societies and panels. But Nigel Cameron is not asking for the resurgence of ecumenical and thoughtful theologians and religionists like H. Richard Niebuhr, quiet leader of what would become the entire generation of leaders in Christian ethics for almost a century. But many of them wouldn't share the view that secularism in bioethics is an evil, or even that it took things "off the religious track." Many of the leading religious bioethicists, for example, took issue with the Catholic establishment's incredible position that a patient who had essentially no brain, and had been in a vegetative state for years, Terry Schiavo, should be kept on life support forever. Like Prof. John Paris, SJ, arguably the leading Catholic scholar in bioethics, who ripped into the position of the Church – on the Church's own doctrinal grounds. I doubt seriously that the Center for Bioethics and Human Dignity, Trinity International University, or Nigel Cameron's new think tank will be making a hire of John Paris.

When Nigel Cameron says that Christians are losing bioethics, it is a call to arms. He's smart, and he leads a movement that is on the fast track to allying with the neoconservatives (led by Leon Kass of the University of Chicago, former campaigner and bioethics commission chair for President Bush) and the purists (led by Carl Elliot, professor at the University of Minnesota). He'll get his think tank – in fact you could argue that Leon Kass' big booster, the American Enterprise Institute, is well on the way to playing that role. And check out the awfully slick and relatively new right-wing bioethics web site: bioethics.com, as well as their journal

Ethics & Medicine: A Christian Perspective, which can't (and doesn't) lay the claim to having its articles peer reviewed by secular scholars (it just uses a name that suggests as much). Even in a democratic administration, politicized bioethics that casts aspersions at mainstream bioethics, a peer-reviewed field in every sense, as though a bunch of liberals are taking the counsel of corporate whores and atheists and nothing more, has, one might hope, a fading visage.

Case 56   Pharma Owns Bioethics (and Other Fables)

Writes Carl Elliot in the *Lancet*:[2]

> North American bioethics has a growing credibility problem. As the influence of bioethics has grown, so has the willingness of bioethicists to seek out funding from the pharmaceutical and biotechnology industries. These industries have begun to fund bioethics centres, lectureships, consultants, advisory panels, conferences, and private regulatory boards. The results of this industry-funded work are now making their way into peer-reviewed academic journals. Readers of the medical and bioethics literature have recently seen articles on the ethics of recruiting homeless individuals for research, funded by Eli Lilly; on the ethics of biotechnology and the developing world, funded by Glaxo, Merck, and Pfizer; on the ethics of stem-cell research, funded by Geron; and the ethics of placebo-controlled trials for mood-altering drugs, funded by antidepressant manufacturers. They have also seen pharma-funded university bioethicists collaborating on ethics articles with biotech entrepreneurs and a medical ethics and humanities journal issue funded by a pharmaceutical lobbying organisation. The authors of these articles have disclosed their industry ties, but readers are left to wonder: is an industry-funded bioethicist a bioethicist that we can trust?
>
> Even discussions of conflict of interest have become tainted by questions of conflict of interest – or at least the perception of a potential conflict. The *American Journal of Bioethics* recently published an article on the ethics of taking gifts from the pharmaceutical industry which was itself funded by Pfizer, while the American Medical Association's Council on Ethics and Judicial Affairs launched an educational project on industry gifts that was funded by a $675,000 gift from the pharmaceutical industry. When the US National Institute of Health (NIH) commissioned a so-called blue-ribbon panel to investigate their conflict-of-interest scandal, in which researchers were found to have undisclosed financial ties to private industry, the blue-ribbon panel included an insurance executive, the vice-president of a for profit healthcare company, the chief executive officer of a leading weapons

manufacturer, and the director of the Ethics Resource Center, Washington, D.C., an ethics institute funded by Merck. One can see the reasoning behind appointing these panelists, but they are hardly likely to inspire trust in observers worried that the NIH has become too close to private industry.

I'm sure Pfizer is just thrilled with the "ethics of taking gifts" publication that Elliot lambasts (here and elsewhere) published in *The American Journal of Bioethics*. What pharmaceutical company doesn't want to be identified as funding a study that finds that pharma's most frequent marketing practice, one in which it itself engages, is pervasive and unethical, and then to see that publication in a major journal and splashed all over most US newspapers? And then to become the foundation of a policy that has kicked pharma reps out of medical schools almost entirely?

It is becoming clear that Dr. Elliot is trying to cause rather than report on a scandal about industry funding of bioethics. There is a scandal to report on – bioethics is being compromised – but the powerful who are taking over bioethics are not in the world of industry but in politics. There is a well-developed neoconservative bioethics "movement" now, a virtually unadulterated tool of the last presidential administration that has recently busied itself with apologetics for the Bush administration position on stem cell research.

Meanwhile, there is no evidence whatsoever that bioethics is becoming a "thought leader" tool for industry, a shill, or a marketing device. Elliot's lists of who is taking what money are (ironically) just flat wrong, poorly researched to the point that they are worthy of Sen. George McCarthy. His post office pictures of the 10 most wanted, above, lack any context and show a genuine disregard for the truth. I for one have tired of reading one accusation after another about the way in which my colleagues are bought by industry, while Elliot utterly ignores the way in which pharma funds virtually every institution in which bioethics is practiced – and more important ignores the bigger threat to "buying bioethics" that comes almost exclusively from the right wing. I for one am very proud of the work I and others in bioethics have done in the context of funding by industry, and I am convinced that much of it was possible – and that it was possible for my colleagues and I to challenge industry so pointedly – exactly because we had that funding. Moreover, I think the fact that industry is willing to pay to have its own practices examined is a sign of progress, and it seems arcane bordering on mindless to suggest that a line must be drawn between Michael Moore's *Capitalism* and the holy temple of academia.

121

Elliot makes innumerable claims that strain credibility about the erosion of bioethics' integrity among the general public, and the biggest problem with them is the assertion that there is a growing wariness about industry bioethics. However, to the extent that it is true that there is wariness about bioethics and industry, that wariness is almost certainly a product of Elliot's own well-placed articles in which he alleges it to be true. For example, in speeches Elliot has taken to describing a speech at Minnesota by Alan Milstein, the attorney who has built a major practice in litigating against institutions (including Penn) that have been alleged to be involved in research misconduct. Milstein, Elliot says, mentioned in his speech that he was proud of having sued bioethicists (by which he meant that he named one bioethicist, Arthur Caplan, in a lawsuit against Penn involving the case of young Jessie Gelsinger's death while enrolled in gene therapy). The big punchline in Carl's talk is that, "to my great surprise, amazingly," the crowd broke out into applause at the mention of suing bioethicists. With embarrassment, Elliot says it: people are beginning to clap when they hear that we bioethicists are being sued, because we're all bought out, tools of industry. But I went back and got the tape: the rousing applause for suing bioethicists? It simply did not happen. A couple of people (2) laughed and clapped twice, no doubt because the idea of suing their former colleague Art Caplan, who made it possible there would even be a major bioethics center at Minnesota, was pretty laughable. Draw your own conclusions: the tape is online at the University of Minnesota. My point is that Elliot doesn't let facts get in the way.

The cautionary tale Elliot spins in the *Lancet*, enough to inspire an early online publication of this article, and tons of media interest, is interesting and grounded in an important concern about academic integrity, but it isn't as simple as Elliot makes it out to be. Elliot, whose hard money position at Minnesota is funded in large part (as are most bioethics positions in major medical centers) by dollars from pharmaceutical companies directly to the medical school, is searching for a monastic cleanliness of funding that simply doesn't exist. And he preys on the all-too-easy trick of attracting criticism to ethicists on the grounds that they violate ethics, rather than arguing for ways in which ethics and industry can co-exist.

The most revered institutions of bioethics during its early years, like the Hastings Center, received and receive huge, and at times majority, contributions from industry. Elliot's answer? Well, they wouldn't survive otherwise. . .and academic Centers have a choice. In Elliot's world there are villains and heros and indulgences for the heros.

122

There are big issues here that deserve to be treated with much more subtlety and far less conspiracy theory. The notion that bioethics is losing its credibility has become a self-fulfilling crusade for Elliot, who seems to be waging an almost single handed campaign to convince a broad audience that bioethics is less than credible, rather than (as he claims) reporting on the evolving demise of the field.

I'm sympathetic to the quest – my own resignation as chair of the ethics advisory board of Advanced Cell Technology started this whole mess in the media in the first place, inspiring calls by the media and then by Elliot himself, who began in the article about my resignation to refer to the difference between guard dogs and lap dogs. I was lucky enough to be a guard dog, I guess. For a few minutes. But those of us who are worried about the dangers of corporate influence on ethics need to direct our attention to best practices rather than identifying villains. It is time for those who claim to want a better bioethics to abandon Elliot's McCarthyism.

The reporters are calling. They keep asking the same question: is industry funding changing the claims or orientation or bearing or credibility of bioethics? I try again and again to think of a single point at which that might even seem to have happened. But, nope, none appear. Except for that one, glaring set of examples: huge funding from the religious right to keep a PVS patient in Florida alive at all costs – bioethics paid for by the right wing of the Republican Party. But hey, that Terri Schiavo thing had no real impact, except on a few hundred million viewers worldwide. Let's focus on a dozen small grants to two or three bioethics centers and see if any ethicists have been "bought." Or maybe not.

Case 57   The Kevorkianization of Cloning

The wrong way to approach scientific innovation of great public import is to throw it like a pie into the face of the unprepared public.

Since the cloning of Dolly the sheep, research involving nuclear transfer-derived cells – and intelligent debate about that research – has been plagued by a phenomenon you might call "kevorkianization." Whatever your view of physician-assisted suicide, the now-late and legendary convicted felon Jack Kevorkian was the last person on earth who should have been the public advocate for the procedure. Dropping off cadavers in a rusty Volkswagen van on the way to press conferences, he turned euthanasia into reality TV, extolling wisdom about the wishes and conditions of his "patients "and promoting a chain of euthanasia shops.

Kevorkian's untimely decision to make theater out of coping with suffering at the end of life resulted in the total collapse of public discussion about the national need to improve hospice care, nursing homes, and Medicare. To this day, far more attention has been focused on assisted suicide in Oregon than on the medication coverage for the elderly or on palliative care at the end of life.

And so it has been with the manipulation and engineering of cells. In February 1997, Ian Wilmut kevorkianized nuclear transfer. First, he elected to label the most revolutionary and complex exercise of human procreative control in history as "cloning," conjuring up inaccurate images of a Xerox machine that would yield two, say, Kate Beckinsales. Worse, the first "clone" was named after Dolly Parton, the well-endowed country music singer, because the embryo was engineered in part from adult sheep mammary cells.

Wilmut gave his first press conferences unprepared to face questions about why anyone would birth a mammal using nuclear transfer without first holding, at a minimum, an ethical discussion about the implications for humans and agriculture. He was clearly horrified by the subsequent misuse of the word cloning by the media, and was the first to embrace the harried explanations by bioethicists that a cloned human wouldn't be an actual copy.

But the sheep had already been labeled. The world went nuts in a mad rush to ban everything remotely related to nuclear transfer. Efforts to keep discourse civil in the wake of the naming of "clones" were made even more difficult by the parade of lunatics who wanted to make one. Remember the UFO cult, the Raelians, and physicist Richard Seed? Later, that sensationalism has been somewhat quieted by the steady flow of information about the agricultural and medical benefits of cloning.

Scientists such as Wilmut were leaders once it became clear how to lead. He was quick to say that human cloning would be wrong, and he and I actually coauthored an approach to regulating human cloning to help in that effort. But have other high-profile members of the scientific community learned from early mistakes with euthanasia and cloning that the wrong way to approach scientific innovation of great public import is to throw it like a pie into the face of the unprepared public? I'm not so sure.

During the unraveling of Hwang Woo Suk in South Korea, even Wilmut decided that he would seize the moment to make a very public start of making cloned human embryos, and publishing a book in which he reverses himself on his previous moral objections by embracing

124

reproductive cloning. The timing is doubly bad for the public's perception of cloning, because Wilmut found himself fending off likely unwarranted charges that he had essentially no right to claim authorship in the key scientific paper about Dolly. The anti-abortion, anti-stem cell research crowd could not have designed a more effective PR perfect storm.

Wilmut has said that he is as disconcerted by Hwang's dishonesty, just as he was by the media's misconstrual of the word clone. But that isn't the point. Whether controversial researchers call on ethicists and others to help them think about how to frame, conduct, and report on research can make all the difference. Scientists who will be putting human neuronal cells into the brains of mice cannot for a minute believe that the public will be satisfied by the assurance that something so radical has as its sole fail-safe that scientists will look out for any signs that the mice are "acting human." Those who put cellular engineering into action in agriculture, medicine, and nanotechnology must begin with the recognition that the "embryonic stem cell research debate" has become, with gay marriage, one of the two most powerful political debates of the decade, drawing attention, money, and strategic planning away from so much amazing potential in tissue engineering. Stem cell researchers and tissue engineers who would rush to market with test tube beef or rush to clinical trials with artificial organs should take a minute to study the lessons of Dr. Death.

Case 58   Not in the Bush Leagues Anymore

With his August 9, 2001 address regarding stem cell research, President Bush rose to an impossible challenge. Watching the President talk about his dinner table conversations and his private anguish over stem cell research (which we now know thanks to his autobiography was facilitated in significant part by Leon Kass, PhD, who would come to lead his bioethics council), I found myself amazed. Rather than fumbling through his speech as so many of unexpected, he rose to the occasion, doing a laudable job of explaining the intricacies involved in both stem cell research in general and his decision in specific.

The problem with the Bush compromise is that while it was masterful statesmanship, it was bad policy.

First, the Bush policy limited the federal funding of research on stem cells to a tiny number of stem cell "lines" – the figure of 60 floated by the media after his speech turned out in reality to be closer to one-third of that number. That meant that under Bush's funding policy, the nearly $250 million for stem cell research in the first year of the federal funding program would be insulated from the controversial practice of destroying embryos to derive the cells. And that, in turn, meant that the thousands and thousands of embryos that were destined to be destroyed by freezing, that have been frozen so long that they could never be used for any kind of embryo adoption, simply were discarded. Opportunity lost, nothing gained.

By President Bush's own logic – namely that the tragedy of a lost embryo should result in some good – the frozen embryos should have been used, if only so that the research done could come to the best possible good and the embryos truly are not destroyed in vain. But that is logic that never crossed the president's mind or his desk.

Second, President Bush's compromise pads the wallet of a few – perhaps only one or two – companies. A large percentage of the revenue that came from federally funded research on existing stem cell lines ended up paying for these companies' patents on stem cell research. This hardly seems in the spirit of federally funding research – to the corporate interests go all the spoils.

While the nations of the world have been mulling the issue of funding stem cell research, these small companies used venture capital to push ahead. Former Governor of Wisconsin and former Secretary of Health and Human Services, Tommy Thompson, helped to create the most important owner of this research, the University of Wisconsin Alumni Research Foundation (WARF).

WARF may literally own all of those existing cell lines Bush refers to- and may stand to build a research empire from the royalties and "reach through agreement" that ensures that it owns essentially anything created from its cells.

If embryos discarded after IVF had been used, Wisconsin would have made little from stem cell research. Instead, under Bush policy, a tariff must be paid for any stem cell research.

It neither looked good, nor was it good public policy. It set a bad precedent for the ownership of basic science by small companies.

No more stumbling

While the polling data suggested President Bush's position was out of sync with the views of most Americans in 2001, the president set a good tone during his speech that Thursday night. This was not the George W. Bush who lost the popular vote to Vice President Al Gore or who stumbled on the campaign trail when asked about his plan for treating degenerative diseases, mumbling about a "plan to stop Alzheimer's."

Watching President Bush discuss what is arguably the most important research challenge of the new century, I found myself believing I was watching President Clinton. President Bush has in fact duplicated the policy of President Clinton, which was to allow some stem cell research but to distinguish stem cell lines from the embryos that produce them. President Bush out-Clintoned Clinton: he portrayed his compromise on the funding of stem cell research as an anguished defense of family values. Even Jerry Falwell, noted fundamentalist Christian opponent of abortion, had to concede that he saw Bush's comments as a sign of integrity. Not compromise, not wishy-washy dissembling Integrity.

President Clinton and Vice President Gore, and their political appointees in the Department of Health and Human Services and National Institutes of Health, used the same position as a way to avoid criticism by pretending that no embryos were to be destroyed.

But President Bush bit the bullet and acknowledged that stem cells have been made from the destruction of embryos, and that the destruction of embryos should not be in vain. Note the difference.

Liberals argued that it is a mistake to let embryos in the freezer go to waste. President Bush argued that the destruction of embryos must be a last alternative and that embryo adoption would be better, but that ultimately stem cell research – perhaps with stem cells from adults or discarded placentas – must be investigated.

Nor did President Bush opt for hype. Where young Bill Clinton made compromises by touting the amazing advantages of his policy, President Bush opted instead to point out the failings of fetal research and the importance of moving ahead slowly.

He chose a conservative to head a board that would direct stem cell research under the presidency. But unlike President Clinton he gave the board real power and responsibility and indicated that there would be broad and bipartisan representation, which unfortunately turned out not to be the case.

We expected Bush to stammer through a speech. Instead, he proved himself a statesman. His rhetoric was not that of an isolationist who would single out the United States against the world, but rather that of a person who has listened in a genuine way and accomplished what he always identified as his gubernatorial Texan skill: the uniting of the parties.

It will be difficult for Democrats to be partisan in their reaction to President Bush because, as has been the case since the mid-1970s, the monopoly on discussion of family values seems to belong to the Republicans, including the newly eloquent George Bush.

Curse of the times

The curse of interesting times plagued the stem cell research debate in 2001. It was a very exciting time in science, yet frought with uncertainty and hope. The key was wisdom, cautious progress and optimism.

The debate continues well into the Obama administration, whose policy on federal funding of embryonic research extended just a few inches beyond what Bush's did. If stem cell research produces new advances in the coming years we will be here again, discussing the question of how far to go.

The compromise was not what many US scientists hoped for. President Bush's veto and his executive power put an end to another stem cell policy which many had hoped would allow the United States to lead the world in stem cell research. But many of those concerns quickly faded away as states took up the slack that the federal government gave. These efforts in the state vastly outstrip the efforts by the federal government, even in the Obama presidency, and will likely be the fact that prevents a "brain drain" in stem cell research for years to come.

Case 59   Professor Hurlbut, Your 15 Minutes Are Up

The Culture of Life Foundation reported on the news that the stem cell debate will soon be "solved":

> A member of the President's Council on Bioethics believes he may have found a way to obtain stem cells with the same potential as embryonic stem cells without creating or destroying a human embryo.[3]

At last, a brilliant idea for getting around the big problem with embryonic stem cell research. It came from President's Council on Bioethics member William Hurlbut, who constantly complained that those who favor embryonic stem cell research are – his term – "not morally serious" enough. But he had his idea vetted by "prominent Catholic clerics and other ethicists," to see if the technology he proposes is morally acceptable. The idea? The pro-life newsletter gushes:

> in Hurlbut's method the gene responsible for creating the placenta is turned off. Hurlbut contends that this prevents an embryo from ever being created. But like traditional cloning, the egg still generates inner cell mass, or the "blank" cells, that some scientist believe have the greatest research potential. The [Boston] *Globe* reports that parts of the technique are currently being performed on mice.

Sounds great, right? It even sounds oddly familiar, probably. That is because it has been proposed in several forms by at least a dozen scientists who actually work in the area, and published in (among other places) *Nature*, although not by Hurlbut. But Hurlbut thinks his solution is important and scientifically significant, and conservatives are everywhere trumpeting the significant scientific breakthrough.

There's just one problem with taking Hurlbut at face value: He has no publications in stem cell biology, ethics, theology, or any part of clinical IVF. Nor is he, an MD, in clinical practice in that or any other area. Stanford faculty who have asked the president of that institution to release him have pointed out that he has allowed and personally encouraged the description of Hurlbut as a "Stanford scientist."

Hurlbut based the moral utility of his claim on the fact that he vetted it with priests.

The *Boston Globe* covered his theory, and right to lifers are beside themselves with joy at the morally serious solution. (Actually, some of the pro-life leaders are beginning to see the fix Hurlbut's idea puts them in.) But there are many, many problems with Hurlbut's claims that even a visit to the Pope won't fix:

1. He makes assumptions about what counts as an embryo, a matter on which no ten embryo researchers agree,
2. He thus makes assumptions about when the destruction of embryonic material would count as destruction of an embryo, a person, or a human life for either scientists or clerics,
3. He makes no effort whatever to describe why his proposal is somehow less objectionable than other nuclear transfer technologies that he has campaigned against so vigorously.

Soon after, the *Washington Post* reported that Hurlbut's idea was mocked by a visiting scientist at the council, but that nonetheless the council is trading on the prominence afforded to it by Hurlbut's "big ticket idea," and as a direct result Leon Kass, chair of the Bush President's Council on Bioethics, did in fact hold hearings on "solutions" to the stem cell problem, which (surprisingly to me, anyway) were hailed by Kass himself as important stuff.[4] One might have guessed that Kass would be a bit embarrassed that his handpicked council would advance ideas as potentially repugnant (following his analysis in his own writing) as Hurlbut's, designed to sidestep rather than engage a debate. Yet, Kass does try his best to make the ideas sound thoughtful:

> Kass said the ideas raise the possibility that "the partisans of scientific progress and the defenders of the dignity of nascent human life can go forward in partnership without anyone having to violate things they hold dear."[5]

But the idea is neither an artful dodge nor a successful one.

Congressmen really are dumb enough to believe William Hurlbut

I really believed that the 15 minutes were over. How wrong I was. Roscoe, Rick and Phil held an actual briefing for Congressional staff to discuss how to do embryonic stem cell research without harming embryos. Altered nuclear transfer (ANT), which we prefer to call semantic nuclear transfer to signify that it is stupid nonsense, is going to be all the rage. And Hurlbut, who seems to have acquired something approximating an academic title in Stanford's Neurosciences Institute, helped brief the crowd on the technique we have discussed on this blog ad nauseam:

> Dr. William Hurlbut is a physician and a Consulting Professor in the Neuroscience Institute at Stanford. He is a member of the President's Council on Bioethics and the author of Altered Nuclear Transfer, one of the four proposals for a solution to our stem cell impasse discussed in the Council's White Paper. Altered Nuclear Transfer would employ the basic technology of nuclear transfer (SCNT) but with an alteration such that no embryo is created, yet pluripotent stem cells (the functional equivalent of embryonic stem cells) are produced. The scientific feasibility of this technique has been established in mouse models by stem cell biologist Rudolf Jaenisch at MIT. Recent advances in developmental biology suggest promising prospects for this approach and it has received wide support among leading moral philosophers and religious authorities.[6]

Dr. Hurlbut is a strong proponent of legislation to fund these proposals and in a Senate hearing last July described them as providing "one small island of unity in a sea of controversy." At the briefing Dr. Hurlbut said, "Approaches, such as these, that open scientific progress while preserving the most fundamental moral principles, are in the best spirit of positive pluralism and would be a triumph for our nation as a whole."

I swear, this guy should run for office; with so many red states to choose from, surely someone needs a neoconservative willing to lie this blatantly about stem cell research.

The high watermark of Hurlbut

Florida Gov. Jeb Bush decided to give loads of credence to our favorite neocon William Hurlbut's bogus theory that embryonic stem cells can be derived from what the right-to-life folks have described as "handicapped embryos." Notably, it went down in flames in Massachusetts after being embraced by Mitt Romney there.

But *Wired* magazine has something invested in Hurlbut, having published what amounts to a puff piece about him in May 2005, and in so doing having essentially been suckered into what is becoming a hilarious snake-oil road show. Orchestrated by Hurlbut, but gaining momentum as it acquires signatures, this is a bit like Jeremy Rifkin's zillion signature petition in the late 1990s against gene patenting, in that it is being signed by folks who will later realize what they are signing and come to regret it.

The best evidence of this of course is the fact that no significant stem cell researcher will give Hurlbut the time of day, nor have any senior scientists said anything about the Hurlbut proposal other than "who is that guy, again?"

In any event, Governor Bush, who lends considerable expertise in bioethics, particularly in end-of-life issues, opines that Hurlbut is the "bright person" who can solve the big ethics problem about stem cell research:

> "I think taking of human life to create life is a huge contradiction morally," Bush said. "But . . . there are other really bright people in this issue who share that view who are trying to find an alternative that would not retard the advancement of science."[7]

Jeb Bush's solution to the stem cell problem, The Hurlbut Suggestion, or semantic nuclear transfer, as we refer to it, prompted the New York *Times*' Gina Kolata to essentially break the embargo on a major science journal's publication of studies that show, well, something we can't write down yet about how some folks have achieved success in producing embryonic cells that promise to anger nobody, by using techniques that make embryonic cells without awakening the Torquemadas of the right.

The research all stems, Kolata claims, from his brilliant idea that we could avoid the embryonic stem cell debate if we could just make little embryo-like things that are somehow disabled enough (through the prior alteration of the adult somatic cell from which they derive) that their creation will not involve the potential for birth. It seems to us to be a cross between nuts and a smokescreen, and the idea has (we noted) not really persuaded folks from the world of right to life either.

If having read all of our discussion and incessant whining about the idiocy of these "almost an embryo, but not" ideas you are still thirsty for more, then don't wait another moment, surf on over right now to read Ms. Kolata's "Hunting for Ways Out of an Impasse" at the *New York Times* site.

Language matters

Even the conservative *Dallas Morning News* couldn't resist mocking Washington ethicist-in-chief Tom DeLay's use of the phrase "dismemberment of embryos" to describe stem cell research. The paper went looking for debate about whether or not DeLay was in some sense justified for describing stem cell research as a deliberate torture and slaughter of little people. But what's to discuss? Nobody could defend the choice of "dismemberment" as a metaphor to describe embryonic stem cell research, right? Well, there is one guy who will. Just when I was ready to believe he might not be completely without shame, I read:

> William Hurlbut, a Stanford University bioethicist who sits on the Pre-sident's Council on Bioethics, defended Mr. DeLay's description. "The point he is trying to get at is conceptually correct. He is trying to make vivid the realization that even though they are very tiny, they are integrated organisms, not 'inchoate clumps of cells' as some scientists have mislead-ingly said," Dr. Hurlbut said. ". . . the truth is that even though it is very tiny, the blastocyst-stage embryo from which ES [embryonic stem] cells are harvested does have distinct parts. To disaggregate it to get the ES cells is to pull apart a human body in its incipient but unfolding form."[8]

Yes, Mr. Hurlbut, I'm sure Rep. DeLay worked hard dumbing down his sophisticated sense of embryonic dismemberment, and was only "trying to make vivid the realization that even though they are very tiny, they are integrated organisms, not "inchoate clumps of cells." Just checking, but

132

did DeLay work on his position about "inchoate clumps of cells" while he was riding in some corporate jet? Or maybe it was while he was up late at night worrying about Terry Schiavo? I'll give you $50,000 if you can find a single instance of Tom DeLay using the word inchoate in a sentence. Though I am sure that he has given the deepest of thought to stem cell research. Ethics are on his mind.

Lakoff's fellow linguist Deborah Tannen has another interesting interpretation of the rationale for DeLay's comment, one not hatched (like Hurlbut's) on the moon:

Deborah Tannen, a Georgetown University linguistics professor, said that by using the word dismemberment, Mr. DeLay and others opposed to embryonic stem cell research are trying to associate it with the controversial late-term abortion, which critics also refer to as "partial-birth" abortion.

"That was such a successful campaign because it gave the impression that they were dismembering a child," Dr. Tannen said. "They are trying to create an association with babies, and they want to push it back earlier and earlier. I guess stem cells would be the extreme of that, but they're just cells. In order to dismember something, it has to have limbs, and cells don't have limbs."[9]

So, oddly, the question of language has become front burner in the stem cell debate. *New York Times* science writer Gina Kolata, for example, points out that the uses and abuses of the terms "cloning" and "embryo" in particular have become very important to the debate over stem cells – with both sides arguing that their description of the term is based on science and the other's based on politics, religion or some other such superstition:

cloning opponents are disturbed by the way stem cell scientists these days almost always speak of "somatic cell nuclear transfer" rather than "cloning." "The most important thing to be said is that the language is changing and it seems to have an agenda behind it to make things more acceptable," said Dr. John Kilner, the president for the Center for Bioethics and Human Dignity, which opposes cloning and destroying human embryos to extract their stem cells. "I'm concerned," he added. "People ought to debate the scientific issues on the merits."[10]

Ah yes, the merits.

The truth is that the abuses of the language game are in fact on both sides. I'm not sure that it could ever have seemed truly reasonable to describe the product of a procreative process as a "clump of cells;" the language is truly loaded and deliberately uses science to confuse the listener. However, the abuses of science by proponents of stem cell research pale by comparison to the abuses of the right wing, including many who use their pretentious language to obscure the fact that they have no idea whatsoever what they are talking about:

> Dr. Leon Kass, the [President's Commission on Bioethics'] chairman, argued last week that the South Koreans' feat should not be disguised by jargon. "The initial product of their cloning technique is without doubt a living cloned human embryo, the functional equivalent of a fertilized egg," Dr. Kass wrote in an e-mail message. "If we are properly to evaluate the ethics of this research and where it might lead," he continued, "we must call things by their right names and not disguise what is going on with euphemism or misleading nomenclature." [11]

The silky language doesn't disguise a simple claim: the product of reproductive nuclear transfer is "without doubt a living cloned human embryo, the functional equivalent of a fertilized egg." Find me one stem cell researcher, indeed one embryologist, who would agree that "without a doubt" that is true. Having studied embryologists' perceptions of stem cell research, I can tell you there's no such person out there. Find me a scientist who will speak of the "functional equivalent" of an embryo. Get started now, though, because no scientist has used the language of function in basic biology in fifty years, and because nobody – and I mean nobody – in science would argue that embryos have a clearly defined "function." What would the function of a fertilized embryo be? To develop into a baby. The Korean cells can't.

Both sides of the stem cell debate want to control language – but neither can really claim to have accessed facts or even "scientific reality." In this debate, the politics – resulting in socially accepted language – really will determine the science.

Saletan on Zoloth on Hurlbut on stem cells

In a piece that is just a bit too clever, William Saletan accuses Laurie Zoloth of being a bit too clever. He reviews a dialog between Zoloth and William Hurlbut that took place at a typical forum about stem cell research. The impression he takes from the encounter can be summarized very briefly, although the nuanced "I was there-ness" that Saletan's pieces have taken on will be lost in my summary. Which is not, you will see if you read his new piece, an altogether bad thing.

Saletan points out that Hurlbut's dopey idea (altered nuclear transfer) unraveled under Zoloth's retorts, leaving Hurlbut livid and incoherent. If you read this blog you will find the latter fact easy to believe. Hurlbut, I have argued, has devolved into a charlatan selling a snake-oil science-based solution to the stem cell debate. But he does a fabulous impression of a sincere and devoted scientist who only means well. And, equally, Saletan performs: his act is "the liberal who feels bad for neoconservatives," and when he is in character he writes with a voice that can be quite annoying.

In what seem like a dozen columns for *Slate* it goes like this: he begins his commentary by telling us that he is "sitting in the audience" at events in which the neoconservatives participate, and the message he brings back each time is that although he himself is liberal, the problem with liberals is that they are too cavalier, too loosy-goosy with the facts, and not ... Second ... here it comes ... serious enough.

So the account he gives of this event is all-too-familiar to me as a loyal reader of his new and fairly comprehensive writing about bioethics issues. It amounts to the claim that Zoloth wins the debate but cheats, and not because she is intending to cheat but instead because the overconfidence of liberals leads them to fail to question facts.

The problem with this argument is simple. It is wrong. Zoloth, he claims, had her facts wrong. His example is the question of whether altered nuclear transfer (ANT) will reliably produce an embryo that will not implant. He says that he trusted Zoloth – her authority on the matter as a disputant until she got them wrong:

> At lunch, Zoloth said the idea behind ANT – knocking out a gene called Cdx2 to prevent development of an implantable embryo – wouldn't reliably succeed because gene knockouts produce a range of outcomes. I asked for her evidence that a range of implantation outcomes would occur with Cdx2 deletion. That's how it works, she assured me. But as I write this, I'm looking at the published report on the ANT experiment. It says "none of the Cdx2 [-deleted] nuclear transfer blastocysts formed visible implantation sites (0 out of 40)."[12] There goes my faith.

Well, that is a clever claim to make but all Saletan had to do was look deeper and he would see that while this is the report made in the Nature piece, it does not in any way exhaust the claim Zoloth is making. Her point is not that the group who conducted this single experiment should have found "implantatability" but that work onCdx2 deletion has shown that there are a wide variety of effects on the developing cells that would include some embryos having the potential to be implantable, and that from a pro-life point of view if that potential exists at all, we're killing someone. Her point is subtle and frankly that is what makes me furious. And not with some sort of simple "liberal indignation" of the sort Saletan has begun to assert that liberal bioethicists hold.

So there's the rub. Saletan misses the fact that Hurlbut is at bottom disingenuous, he has heard countless times from many disputants including many of the top biologists in several related fields that his purported solution is voodoo and a political tactic at best. Hurlbut is clearly thrilled that the bad science that under girds the attempts to avoid the stem cell debate has advanced as far as it has, so far in fact that perfectly respectable stem cell researchers are publishing wacky science in *Nature* in order to keep the dogs at bay. Hurlbut, it should be restated in this regard, apparently has no training in ethics, and is not a stem cell researcher. He is the one playing fast and loose, and Saletan should perhaps have taken just a few minutes to identify the multiple claims to that effect in the voluminous literature on such "solutions."

So why, when Zoloth presents cogent arguments that position stem cells in relation to complex social and political phenomena and scientific issues, is Saletan hammering her for that sin?

Simple. He likes the seriousness, the monasticism of the Kass crowd. It is appealing because it feels academic, sincere, earnest. When Hurlbut pleads for us to take things more seriously, to not be "rude," it is because that political – and strictly political – tactic works for him. But when Hurlbut leaves the cathedral, he is flying all over the country on an entrepreneurial mission to kill stem cell research, shows up everywhere he can, and courts profile articles like nobody in the history of bioethics, never once confessing to being an amateur in a field where most folks believe you should actually be a scholar of ethics before professing to be an ethicist.

Saletan is taken in by the claim that moral seriousness is a phenotype, a thing you can see and smell on people when they talk. It isn't. Real moral seriousness comes from thinking and writing carefully, and that is precisely what Hurlbut does not do. In fact with the exception of the one piece in which he argues for cheating the stem cell debate through the theoretical use of ANT, Hurlbut does not as best I can tell write in the field at all. Either field, in fact, stem cells or bioethics. How can you be a morally serious tutor of bioethics if you don't write in the field? This is the problem Saletan misses. It isn't about trust, it's about scholarship. I am quite sure that the folks who trust Saletan enough to have lunch and discuss the issues would prefer he start there, no matter how exciting the performances of bioethics may be.

Conservatives turn on their own

From the very moment that William Hurlbut floated his dramatic new plan to save us all from the terror of destroying frozen embryos it was clear that, as we foretold, the clock had started on his poorly thought-out "work-around" for stem cells: intentionally producing disabled embryos.

True, for a bit it looked like Leon Kass would push Hurlbut's idea into the fore, with his announcement that the president's bioethics commission would be discussing it (and other ideas), and with his subsequent claim that Hurlbut's idea could save us all from having to debate stem cell ethics any longer. Catholic and protestant fundamentalist leaders jumped for joy. But it was only a matter of time before even the "pro-life" community would wake up to realize that embracing Hurlbut's half-baked neoscientific plan meant doing all sorts of things that amount to what they typically term "playing God."

And so, exactly eight days after it showered Hurlbut with adoration for saving the tiny people, the pro-life lobby has officially turned on Professor Hurlbut for crimes against the little embryos. One biologist interviewed for the "hang Hurlbut" piece in LifeSite today puts their indictment of him squarely: "the process would not create an unknown 'new entity,' but a severely disabled, cloned human being." The anti-abortion people even have an excuse for embracing Hurlbut: they were too dizzied by all that complicated science stuff: "Possibly due to the extremely rarified nature of the technical language, few reservations were raised at the meeting, even by the pro-life Catholics present."

No dodging science with the Hurlbut trick

The circle became truly complete as scientists put to rest the idea that Hurlbut has figured out what counts as an embryo. *New England Journal of Medicine* published an editorial, entitled "Altered Nuclear Transfer in Stem-Cell Research: A Flawed Proposal" by Melton, Daley, and Jennings, that reads in part:

> Hurlbut's argument for the ethical superiority of altered nuclear transfer rests on a flawed scientific assumption. He argues, on the basis of supposed insights from systems biology, that it is acceptable to destroy a CDX2

137

mutant embryo but not a normal embryo, because the former has "no inherent principle of unity, no coherent drive in the direction of the mature human form." But these are ill-defined concepts with no clear biologic meaning, and an alternative interpretation would be that embryos lacking CDX2 develop normally until CDX2 function is required, at which point they die. Philosophers may debate these and other interpretations. We see no basis for concluding that the action of CDX2 (or indeed any other gene) represents a transition point at which a human embryo acquires moral status.[13]

Stem cell legislation at risk

A part of me just does not care that yet again the ridiculous theory advanced by the only man more dangerous to stem cell research than Hwang Woo-suk, William Hurlbut, has become again part of the national debate about the funding of stem cell research.

It didn't bug me when Jeb Bush backed Hurlbut's nonsense.

It didn't bug me when Hurlbut used his mind-numbingly stupid theory to defend Tom Delay.

I was not surprised that having been castigated for the theory's stupidity by real scientists on the Hill and in the *New England Journal*, and by basically every serious stem cell researcher in, um, the world, Hurlbut remained unfazed.

I admit to being a tiny bit annoyed that Slate's William Saletan not only dignified Hurlbut's idea but belittled Laurie Zoloth for questioning Hurlbut's science.

But anyone who has not figured out by now that Hurlbut's poorly thought out plan to make handicapped embryos is both disingenuous claptrap and utterly political in nature is probably not going to be persuaded by any sort of arguments to emerge in the upcoming battle on the hill about federal funding for embryonic stem cell research.

So why not be grumpy about a statement from Senator Frist whose support of embryonic stem cell research was the key break against President Bush just months ago – in which he essentially switches sides using the Hurlbut copout:

> "The new science that may involve embryo research but not require destruction of an embryo is tremendously exciting," Senate Majority Leader Bill Frist (R-Tenn.) said recently. "It would get you outside of the boundaries of the ethical constraints."[14]

Simple. Because it does not matter.

The stem cell debate in Washington is over. Whatever pittance that might be won were Democrats and reasonable Republicans to prevail in their push for additional US government spending would pale by comparison to what will be spent in the states.

It would be wonderful to see the US government spend additional dollars on stem cell research. For the price of a day's military activities in Iraq, the US could be at the lead of the most important medical research in the history of the world.

But instead, it seems clear now that cutting edge regenerative medicine is going to happen offshore and in a few enclaves in the US. What Korea didn't kill, those who published these silly "alternative" theories in Nature – none of whom want to use them and their conceptual Godfather William Hurlbut – may have.

Case 60 The Heady Days of Proposition 71: Stem Cell Research in the California Sun

In January 2005, the *San Francisco Chronicle* reported that Robert Klein, real estate magnate and chair of the California Institute for Regenerative Medicine, the Proposition 71-funded master of ceremonies for $3 billion in stem cell research to be doled out beginning in May 2005, has at long last given an interview. In it he discussed the controversy concerning when the money will be given out for stem cell research, and more important the rules that will be used by CIRM to do so.[15]

AP reports that first amendment groups are furious over tight secrecy concerning how $3 billion in tax dollars will be spent. *ContraCostaTimes* reports on "growing" complaints that the stem cell legislation offers too many opportunities to use stem cell money in California to make institutions rich. And it is certainly true that the stakeholders are running the show: "Many of the 29 board members, appointed by the governor and other elected officials to run the agency, represent research universities and the biotech industry, both of which are expected to win millions of dollars worth of grants." [16]

The guidelines are required by Proposition 71, and while it can revise the guidelines that it puts in place now, it needs good guidelines at the outset, not only because of the law but because of swirling controversy in California about the ties of CIRM board members to the institutions that will be asking for money.

So where will these guidelines come from? The National Academies, who have engaged Virginia bioethicist Jonathan Moreno to run a committee on model guidelines for conducting stem cell research.

"It would be better for us all to be on the same page," said Jonathan Moreno, director of a biomedical ethics center at the University of Virginia and co-chair of the National Academies committee. During a telephone interview Wednesday, Moreno said the National Academies' guidelines are expected to be out by April after a final round of outside reviews and revisions. "The committee has been running since August, and people say, 'Gee, you're taking a long time,'" Moreno said. "But this is hard. For academics, this is a breakneck pace."[17]

It will be helpful indeed for California's stem cell funding group to get the Moreno committee report, which will join several other sets of recommendations on how individual states', states collectively, and the nation should pursue specific standards for stem cell research.

But it is difficult to see how any group writing guidelines for national stem cell policy – or even for state and national policy -can cover both the issues inherent in national dilemmas, and the issues present in the states' differing legal, clinical, political, economic, and social situations, and still be finished in eight months.

And in this case, Moreno and his group are being asked to produce a report that does all of this while taking care to address the issues about model guidelines that would be appropriate to the very, very special "California world," with its own behemoth budget and complex allocation issues.

It remains to be seen whether California will create its own ethics group or ethics research division within Proposition 71, and it would be dangerous indeed for the state to avoid doing so. California state stem cell policy might not be something you want -for the long term anyway – to have "phoned in" at the last minute. What Californians really need to do is hire Jonathan Moreno away from Virginia!

Learning the lessons of Hwang? Nope

Zach Hall the president of the California Institute for Regenerative Medicine says that peer review is the key to prevent fraud in stem cell research. Not a new kind of peer review, or a better review of peer review, or more peer review, just peer review. In the *San Francisco Chronicle*, he is asked what will prevent Hwang-style fraud and other bioethics problems in California. His answer?

"Scientists," responded Zach Hall, president of the California Institute for Regenerative Medicine, the funding entity created by Prop. 71. Warning that every industry has the potential for an Enron, Hall touted the American system of peer review as the best way to expose rogue scientists and bad science and to keep research-funding decisions apart from undue political, religious, or geographic influences. "What will not stop this from happening misgovernment oversight," he said.

Not regulations. This from the guy who is giving out the money. Oversight is the key to giving the money out responsibly. It is one of the reasons why we should give government funding in the first place. California has become the standard-bearer for state-based biotechnology research funding. That, I could have argued, is ok. But not if the standard-bearer claims that fraud is best prevented by peer review.

Bioethicists need not apply

Why doesn't California put a bioethicist on its Proposition 71 governing board dealing with the $3 billion to be allocated for stem cell research? University chancellors and presidents are being nominated up and down as schools' and institutes' top guns clamor to be public intellectuals on this big-ticket funding item, no doubt in part to ensure that their shop gets some of the money. The proposition guarantees seats on the board to some institutions (including the five UCal schools), but why in the world can't there be some slots dedicated to bioethics?

No matter what your position on stem cell research, there simply must be a dedicated stem cell ethics expert among the governors. If it weren't so serious a matter, one would have to laugh at the idea that these University and institute administrators are properly trained to think about how and whether to dispense the money and for which studies. It is a question several are beginning to ask anew, echoing concerns from those who opposed Prop 71 but themselves supported hES research. Bioethics in California has always been a developing phenomenon, although the Stanford Center for Biomedical Ethics is arguably among the top programs in the nation. Hopefully at least some of the ballast for deliberations about which programs should be funded will be provided by people in stem cell bioethics in California. But that is a very, very short list of people.

Even more important, California should finally begin to build up some bioethics programs, particularly in the universities that plan to do significant new stem cell research. If the past is any predictor, that will not be easily accomplished in California, where bioethics has just never really

141

taken a foothold in terms of university budgets and powerhouse faculties. There are plenty of good people in bioethics in California, but it is difficult to identify a group of major research centers in bioethics in the state, despite its preeminent place in biotechnology research. Proposition 71 should be the full employment act for California bioethics, to borrow Art Caplan's description of the role ethics money in the Human Genome Project had on bioethics in the 1990s. But if it is business as usual in the most populous state in the nation, bioethics may become an unfunded sport for university CEOs. That would not only hurt bioethics, it would hurt the people of California, who are clearly hoping for a careful, smart use of the $3 billion windfall for stem cells. For them, ethics has to stay in the mix in a serious way.

The Full Employment Act for stem cell research

Well it's out, at last, the first Request for Applications (RFA) for money from the California Institute for Regenerative Medicine (CIRM) and pronounced "SERM." This thing is a monster – $1.25 million a year proposals are being invited for institutions, each one of which could support up to 16 new scholars in stem cell research. And $800,000 and $500,000 for smaller programs. And that's just the start of it – these are just the grants to pay for training new people to work in the field. The big bucks are going to be in support of actual research initiatives. Places like Stanford for example are going to leverage this money to build new buildings for regenerative medicine. This program has been coming since Californians passed Proposition 71, the $3 billion stem cell initiative.

But when you actually look at the thing, it is just a huge amount of money that will go to a select number of institutions.

Is there ethics money? Well, sort of. The programs "will be required to offer at least one course in stem cell biology and disease and a course in the social, legal and ethical implications of stem cell research." And there is a mandate that CIRM "seeks institutions that will promote interaction among trainees from different fields, especially those trained in basic science and clinical medicine." But there's no gigantic ethics pot here, so the money for bioethics and stem cell research, which everybody thinks ought to be front burner, will require that the big schools in California think intelligently about how important it can be for them to include a real ethics program in their applications for stem cell money. And that is going to require that some of us fly out there and sell that idea to UCLA and other places that have virtually no bioethics right now. And you know, it's such a long flight ...

Anyway, anybody with half a brain out there in bioethics has to be scheming to build a bioethics proposal for one of these big center grants – because that could result in the biggest program in the nation in bioethics quite quickly. Oh yeah and that would serve the public interest.

London and Madison hear a great giant sucking sound

They are running scared in Britain. After months of believing their own press about a purported mass exodus of stem cell researchers, there are some pretty scared venture capitalists now in London. *Financial Times'* Clive Cookson delivered a eulogy for the era of mass optimism, complete with lots and lots of quotes from folks proclaiming the proported "brain drain" is now clearly clogged. The UK, by the way, spends just over 25 percent of the annual amount California has just allocated for stem cell research.

Wisconsin Business reports that California's Prop 71 will vacuum up the states stem cell laboratories and researchers. How much will it take to lure James Thomson? One could be cynical about that threat, given that Wisconsin holds so much intellectual property in stem cell research that Wisconsin profits no matter who is doing the work. But business publications are right to worry that Wisconsin could lose its key figures in stem cell research to Prop 71 and to California.

Surround cell

They just can't seem to get the money flowing in California, where $3 billion, which has to seem like a bigger tab with every passing day, continues to essentially be held up by the lingering nuisance suits. So schools are dealing with the problem in different ways. Some are building buildings anyway, a few are actually getting money from the California Institute for Reproductive Medicine through some kind of arrangement I cannot figure out, but most are shaking trees to find ways to move ahead.

And what makes that so amusing to watch is the sort of folks with billions of dollars who live in the parts of California where stem cell research will be concentrated. Take, for example, Ray Dolby, the surround sound guy, who has just given UCSF $16 million to start a stem cell center.

Finally, it is raining stem cell money

California's stem cell research agency, CA Institute for Regenerative Medicine, has unloaded $39.7 million in grants to Stanford, CalTech, USC, and eight of the University of California campuses. The money is all still encumbered by pending litigation concerning Prop 71, but they are giving it out nonetheless. Sort of. Well, they are giving out IOUs, essentially. But the money is coming.

Notes and References

1. Letter by Dr. Nigel Cameron, "How We Lost 'Bioethics'. . . and How We Can Get It Back," June 23, 2005. Accessed at: www.tothesource.org/6_21_2005/6_21_2005_printer.htm.
2. C. Elliot, "Should Journals Publish Industry-funded Bioethics Articles?," *Lancet*, 2005, 366(9483): 422-4. Accessed at: www.thelancet.com/journals/lancet/article/PIIS0140673605667943/fulltext.
3. Culture of Life Foundation, "Controversial Theory Claims to Discover Morally Acceptable Cloning," November 20, 2004, 2(17). Accessed at: http://culture-of-life.org/content/view/209/.
4. D. Brown, "Two Stem Cell Ideas Presented," *Washington Post*, December 4, 2004. Accessed at: http://www.washingtonpost.com/wp-dyn/articles/A33766-2004Dec3_2.html.
5. Ibid.
6. Ibid.
7. K. Philipkoski, "Gov. Bush Eschews Stem Cells," *Wired Magazine*, June 22, 2005. Accessed at: http://www.wired.com/medtech/health/news/2005/06/67968.
8. *Dallas Morning News.* Accessed at: www.dallasnews.com/sharedcontent/dws/news/politics/national/stories/052805dnnatwords.ed9c6fba.html.
9. Ibid.
10. G. Kolata, "Name Games and the Science of Life," *New York Times*, May 29, 2005. Accessed at: www.nytimes.com/2005/05/29/weekinreview/29kolata.html?pagewanted=print.
11. Ibid.
12. W. Saletan, "Technical Knockout: The Overconfidence of Stem Cell Liberals," November 17, 2005. Accessed at: www.slate.com/id/2130493/.
13. Accessed at: www.nejm.org/doi/full/10.1056/NEJMp048348?ck=nck.
14. Ceci Connolly and Rick Weiss, "Stem Cell Legislation at Risk," *Washington Post*, July 8, 2005. Accessed at: www.washingtonpost.com/wp-dyn/content/article/2005/07/08/AR2005070801817.html.

15. Read full text of interview at: www.sfgate.com/cgi-bin/article.cgi?f=/c/a/ 2005/01/13/BAGVGAPL1I1.DTL.

16. Read full text of article at: www.contracostatimes.com/mld/cctimes/news/ 10578954.htm?1c.

17. C. T. Hall, "Guidelines to Precede Stem Cell Grants: Board Chairman Says Ethical Issues Will Be Resolved," *San Francisco Chronicle*, January 13, 2005. Accessed at: www.sfgate.com/cgi-bin/article.cgi?f=/c/a/2005/01/13/BAGV-GAPL1I1.DTL#ixzz1Sa0MsbnN.

Conclusion
Move Slowly and Stay Cool

A Hot and Cold Running Genius

Change agents in bioethics aren't always bioethicists.

Eva Harris won the MacArthur "genius grant" in 1997 for plenty of reasons. As a Pew Scholar in 2001, her bench work on the molecular virology and pathogenesis of dengue virus – specifically, the determinants for viral transmission – was tied purposefully to developing the epidemiological capacity of scientists in developing countries. Harris has helped many aspiring scientists in the developing world. They learn from her to create and sustain programs of bench science "on the cheap." And sometimes, it bears fruit in vaccines and even the promise of translating what might look like rudimentary science into the promise of a cure for the predominant arthropod-borne disease in the world.

Harris' genius, though, is in bioethics, although I find no record that she has ever used the term in her work. That's perhaps not surprising, given how much time bioethics seems to spend on "bad" scientists. I'm ready to tar Harris with the label "ethicist" because of her compulsive goodness. She can't seem to avoid fixating on "the cash value" of her work, and by that I do not mean the literal value she might have extracted from her most noteworthy accomplishment to date – the development of A Low Cost Approach to PCR: Appropriate Transfer of Biomedical Techniques – which brought DNA amplification to labs that could never have used it otherwise. No, for William James, who coined the term as part of the truly

Bioethics for Beginners: 60 Cases and Cautions from the Moral Frontier of Healthcare,
First Edition. Glenn McGee.
© 2012 John Wiley & Sons, Ltd. Published 2012 by John Wiley & Sons, Ltd.

American philosophy of pragmatism, cash value was the cornerstone of ethical science: Science is good, he and John Dewey opined, when it works. Activism on behalf of vulnerable scientists and endangered people is just the sort of translation that scientists in training can point to as ethical genius.

Today Harris runs the Sustainable Sciences Institute in San Francisco, a nonprofit she began with the money awarded through her McArthur prize. The Institute teaches scientists what she calls "knowledge-based" technology transfer. So for DNA amplification, instead of $100 for silica particles, she teaches scientists in the developing world to begin with "a 20-pound bag of ceramic dust for $5 at the hobby store," and thermocycling based on ice, Bunsen burners, and somebody holding a thermometer. A device that costs $10,000 in even its most rudimentary form in the developed world is suddenly within reach of scientists whose entire programs would otherwise be impossible.

Harris spends much time defending her approach and her advocacy. In an interview with the Institute of International Studies at Berkeley, she puts the matter plainly: "In the United States, if you're a scientist and you take a stand, no one will listen to you. It's an incredible thing in this country, where as soon as you become an advocate or take a stand on an issue, you 'lose your objectivity' and people will no longer respect your science … it's quite a slippery path."[1]

At the dawn of exponential improvements in bioinformatics and genetic epidemiology – where vulnerable subjects donate DNA to scientists from wealthy universities, corporations and governments – there can be no question about who will get the first pills and tests. Objectivity isn't part of the equation: every scientist gets a paycheck. And far be it from me to argue that it is unethical for genomic science to spread its benefits incrementally across the world. But in teaching research ethics one points to the exemplars, and of late far too many have distinguished themselves in the public eye through behavior that is just reprehensible.

Eva Harris represents the good in science, the model that brings many if not most scientists to the lab in the first place, just as surely as young physicians imagine that they will one day cure the poor. Geniuses do good science. In Harris' case, this is true in more than both senses of the word.

Science Must Slow Its Speed

Speed kills. This warning is sage advice. Too bad it's confined to motor vehicle operation. It is badly needed in science.

Consider two examples where the desire to race to be first has caused scientists to veer off the road and get into big, big trouble.

In June 2005, Hwang Woo Suk, a veterinary researcher at Seoul National University in South Korea, reported that he had made embryonic stem cells from human embryos derived from 11 people.

Allegations swirled around him for years that he cut corners in his desire to be the first to make stem cells from cloned human embryos. Then it was revealed that Hwang made his embryos from eggs obtained from women working in his lab. That reeked of coercion, since it would be nearly impossible for a young woman in a hierarchical Korean laboratory to say no to a request for her eggs.

The news broke that the breakthrough reported in Hwang's initial paper in the journal *Science* was fraudulent. Key measurements that would definitely prove that the stem cells Hwang said he made came from his cloned embryos now appear to be too good to be true.

Hwang and his group saw an opening when a lack of government funding in the United States kept the best American embryonic stem cell researchers on the sidelines. They ran to get ahead of the world competition. Now it seems they ran so fast they fell down. A colleague of Hwang said the research was falsified. Hwang stood by his research but asked that the Science article be withdrawn because of errors with accompanying photos. Hwang was convicted of breaking multiple Korean laws related to research and served time in prison. Today, he is back at it again – doing stem cell research in Korea. Time will only tell if prison time taught him anything about the importance of following the rules.

A similar story can be told about the French team that conducted the world's first face transplant. Jean-Michel Dubernard of the University of Lyon grafted a nose, chin and mouth taken from brain-dead donor onto a 38-year-old mother of two from Valenciennes in northern France. Dubernard and the French were racing against teams in the United States and England that were also planning face transplants. Again speed seems to have gotten a prominent researcher in big trouble.

British newspapers reported that the reason the recipient needed a face transplant is that she had tried to kill herself. London's *Sunday Times* said the woman acknowledged in a cell phone interview – though she has denied it elsewhere – that she took an overdose of sleeping pills during a fit of depression. As she lay nearly comatose on the floor, her own dog mauled her face.

There were serious concerns that, physically and emotionally, she may not prove up to the challenge of being the world's first face transplant recipient. But there was more. Three months before the operation she seemed to have given a British filmmaker exclusive rights to her story. What motivated her to decide to go ahead with this risky operation? We will almost certainly never know.

Not only did suicide play a role in the life of the recipient, it has now been revealed that the donor used in the operation had committed suicide. So in their haste the French doctors wound up using a donor whose family must have been emotionally devastated when the request came to donate her face.

But the ethical problems did not end there. There was no evidence that the medical team appointed someone to act as the donor family or the recipient family's advocate. When you are asked about whether you want to be involved in the world's first face transplant, it would be morally prudent to have advice from someone who does not care whether you say yes or no.

Certainly a case can be made for face transplants. There are those with oral cancer or burns or injuries for whom no other real option exists. Since the French case, successful face transplants have been performed in the United States and around the world. But, in the race to be first, the French group appears to have given less than adequate thought to who the donor should be, who the recipient should be, and what scientific foundation should have been laid down before trying the surgery.

These publicized scientific firsts prove more questions need to be asked about how fast researchers have been going when they announce their breakthroughs. Requiring answers will necessarily slow the speed at which science advances, and that in many cases is something that will save lives. That is a trade-off that any rational society ought, and must, be willing to make.

Note

1. Interview can be accessed at: http://globetrotter.berkeley.edu/people/Harris/harris-con0.html.

Sources and Credits

The author and publisher gratefully acknowledge the permission granted to reproduce the copyright material in this book.

Case 1

McGee, G. (1999) "The Dangers of Creating Life in the Lab," MSNBC Breaking Bioethics, 12/15/99, www.msnbc.com

Case 2

McGee, G. (2006) "Design: More Intelligent Every Day," *The Scientist*, 20(1): 28

Case 3

McGee, G. (2007) "'Shroom' Science: Safe and Effective?," *The Scientist*, 21(2): 28

Case 4

McGee, G. (2007) "A Robot Code of Ethics," *The Scientist*, 21(5): 28

Case 5

McGee, G. (2007) "No More Periods, Period," *The Scientist*, 21(6): 23

Bioethics for Beginners: 60 Cases and Cautions from the Moral Frontier of Healthcare, First Edition. Glenn McGee.
© 2012 John Wiley & Sons, Ltd. Published 2012 by John Wiley & Sons, Ltd.

Case 6

McGee, G. (2006) "Search Me Not," *The Scientist*, 20(6): 25

Case 7

McGee, G. (2006) "A Bloody Mess," *The Scientist*, 20(8): 24

Case 8

McGee, G. (1999) "Stem Cells: The Goo of Life and the Debate of the Century," MSNBC Breaking Bioethics, 05/24/99, www.msnbc.com

Case 9

McGee, G. (2006) "Lies, Damn Lies . . . and Scientific Misconduct," *The Scientist*, 20(2): 24

Case 10

McGee, G. (2005) "Zerhouni Means Business at NIH," The American Journal of Bioethics Editors' Blog, 02/01/05, http://blog.bioethics.net/2005/02/zerhouni-means-business-at-nih.html

Case 11

McGee, G. (1999) "While You're Here, How about a Spinal Tap?," MSNBC Breaking Bioethics, 5/19/99, www.msnbc.com

Case 12

McGee, G. (1998) "Study Subject or Human Guinea Pig?," MSNBC Breaking Bioethics, 12/10/98, www.msnbc.com

Case 13

McGee, G. (2005) "The New Tuskegee: Exploiting The Poor in Clinical Trials," The American Journal of Bioethics Editors' Blog, 11/05/05, http://blog.bioethics.net/2005/11/the-new-tuskegee-the-poor-exploited-in-clinical-tr/

Case 14

McGee, G. (2006) " Salt in the Wound - Will India Rise up Against the Oppression of Foreign Clinical Trials?" The Scientist, 20(4): 26

Case 15

McGee, G. (2005) "Dr. Hwang and the Bad Apple Theory of Scientific Misconduct," The American Journal of Bioethics Editors' Blog, 12/25/05, http://blog.bioethics.net/2005/12/dr-hwang-and-the-bad-apple-theory-of-scientific-mi/

Case 16

McGee, G. (2001) "Becoming Genomic: Just What Does It Mean Anyway?," MSNBC Breaking Bioethics, 02/10/2001, www.msnbc.com

Case 17

McGee, G. (2004) "Enhancement Comes from Insecurity," The American Journal of Bioethics Editors' Blog, 12/25/05, http://blog.bioethics.net/2004/12/enhancement-comes-from-insecurity/

Case 18

McGee, G. (1999) "Wearing Genes in the Gulf War," MSNBC Breaking Bioethics, 05/05/99, www.msnbc.com

Case 19

McGee, G. (1999) "Tomorrow's Child: Making Babies in the 21st Century," MSNBC Breaking Bioethics, 06/07/99, www.msnbc.com

Case 20

McGee, G. (2001) "An Argument against Human Cloning," MSNBC Breaking Bioethics, 01/24/2001, www.msnbc.com

Case 21

McGee, G. (1998) "Two Genetic Moms: High-tech Trouble or Double The Love?," MSNBC Breaking Bioethics, 10/28/98, www.msnbc.com

Case 22

McGee, G. (1999) "Grave Robbing the Cradle," MSNBC Breaking Bioethics, 04/08/99, www.msnbc.com

Case 23

McGee, G. (2000) "Baby Banking," MSNBC Breaking Bioethics, 03/22/00, www.msnbc.com

Case 24

McGee, G. (2005) "Cash Strapped American Infertility Docs Cry Out for Mercy," The American Journal of Bioethics Editors' Blog, 01/26/2005, http://blog.bioethics.net/2005/01/cash-strapped-american-infertility-docs-cry-out-fo/

Case 25

McGee, G. (2006) " "Nanoethics": The ELSI of 21st Century Bioethics?," The American Journal of Bioethics Editors' Blog, 01/29/2006, http://blog.bioethics.net/2006/01/nanoethics-the-elsi-of-21st-century-bioethics/

Case 26

McGee, G. (2007) "The Devil and the Deep Blue Sea," *The Scientist*, 21(11): 33

Case 27

McGee, G. (1999) "The Merging of Man and Machine," MSNBC Breaking Bioethics, 01/20/99, www.msnbc.com

Case 28

McGee, G. (2007) "The Devil and the Deep Blue Sea," *The Scientist*, 21(12): 33

Case 29

McGee, G. and McGee, S. J. (2007) "Has the Spread of HPV Vaccine Marketing Conveyed Immunity to Common Sense?," *The American Journal of Bioethics*, 7(7): 1-2

Case 30

McGee, G. (2000) "Is the New Cigarette a Smoking Gun? Eclipse Unethical, Unregulated Research," MSNBC Breaking Bioethics, 04/19/2000, www. msnbc.com

Case 31

McGee, G. (1999) "Universal" Healthcare: A Long Way Off," MSNBC Breaking Bioethics, 02/17/99, www.msnbc.com

Case 32

McGee, G. (2006) "Newborn Screening with a Twist," The American Journal of Bioethics Editors' Blog, 08/06/2006, http://blog.bioethics.net/2006/08/newborn-screening-with-twistunproven.html

Case 33

McGee, G and Caplan, A. (2006) "HIV Testing Must Be Routine," Albany Times-Union, 05/21/2006

Case 34

McGee, G and Caplan, A. (2005) "Re-creating Flu: A Recipe for Disaster," Albany Times-Union, 10/23/2005

Case 35

McGee, G and Caplan, A. (2006) "Pandemic Influenza Requires Trust in Government, Health Care," Albany Times-Union, 02/19/2006

Case 36

McGee, G. (2007) "A Hostile Environment for Environmental Protection Documents," *The Scientist*, 21(3): 26

Case 37

McGee, G. (2007) "Thanks, Andrew Speaker," *The Scientist*, 21(7): 26

Case 38

McGee, G. (1999) "Medicine Is Not a Steel Mill," MSNBC Breaking Bioethics, 06/24/1999, www.msnbc.com

Case 39

McGee, G. (2001) "Does Your Doctor Have Skeletons? Good Luck Finding Them," MSNBC Breaking Bioethics, 05/30/2001, www.msnbc.com

Case 40

McGee, G. (2000) "Medicine's Dirty Laundry," MSNBC Breaking Bioethics, 01/13/00, www.msnbc.com

Case 41

McGee, G. (2000) "Economics and Net Medical Ethics," MSNBC Breaking Bioethics, 06/23/00, www.msnbc.com

Case 42

McGee, G. (2005) "Notinourhospitalyoudont.com," The American Journal of Bioethics Editors' Blog, 02/17/2005, http://blog.bioethics.net/2005/02/noti-nourhospitalyoudontcom.html

Case 43

McGee, G. (2006) "A Health System with Miracles," The American Journal of Bioethics Editors' Blog, 03/23/2006, http://blog.bioethics.net/2006/03/health-system-with-miracles.html

Case 44

McGee, G. (2001) "Redefining Retirement: Beyond Rest and Recreation," MSNBC Breaking Bioethics, 09/09/2001, www.msnbc.com

Case 45

McGee, G. (1999) "The Dangers of Creating Life in the Lab," MSNBC Breaking Bioethics, 12/15/99, www.msnbc.com

Case 46

McGee, G. (1999) "The Fight to Die Well," MSNBC Breaking Bioethics, 06/04/99, www.msnbc.com

Case 47

McGee, G. (1999) "The Case of the Body Snatchers," MSNBC Breaking Bioethics, 12/15/99, www.msnbc.com

Case 48

McGee, G. "A Few Conclusions from the Terri Schiavo Case" appeared in part on blog.bioethics.net, various dates

Case 49

McGee, G. (2006) "Living Wills Save Money? Dude, Did You Really Say That Out Loud?," The American Journal of Bioethics Editors' Blog, 05/26/2006, http://blog.bioethics.net/2005/01/cash-strapped-american-infertility-docs-cry-out-fo/

Case 50

McGee, G. (2006) "The Plural of Anecdote is Not Ambien," *The Scientist*, 20(10): 30

Case 51

McGee, G. (1999) "Fat in America," MSNBC Breaking Bioethics, 08/25/99, www.msnbc.com

Case 52

McGee, G. (1999) "Breakfast for Thought," MSNBC Breaking Bioethics, 09/23/99, www.msnbc.com

Case 53

McGee, G. (2007) "Want Fish? Ethics First, Please," *The Scientist*, 21(1): 26

Case 54

McGee, G. (2005) "Dying for Food." The American Journal of Bioethics 5(2):W1

Case 55

McGee, G. (2005) "Bioethics for Christians, Corporate Whores, and Atheists," The American Journal of Bioethics Editors' Blog, 08/21/2005 http://blog. bioethics.net/2005/08/are-christians-losing-bioethics-to-corporate-whore/

Case 56

McGee, G. (2005) "Pharma Owns Bioethics [and Other Fables]," The American Journal of Bioethics Editors' Blog, 07/05/2005 http://blog.bioethics.net/2005/ 07/pharma-owns-bioethics-and-other-fables.htmlchristians-losing-bioethics-to-corporate-whore/

Citation from *The Lancet* originally appeared in Elliot C. "Should Journals Publish Industry-Funded Bioethics Articles?" The Lancet, Volume 366, Issue 9483, Pages 422 - 424, 30 July 2005 http://www.thelancet.com/journals/lancet/article/ PIIS0140673605667943/fulltext

Case 57

McGee, G. (2006) "The Kevorkianization of Cloning." The Scientist 20(9): 26

Case 58

McGee, G. (2001) "Not in the Bush Leagues Anymore," MSNBC Breaking Bioethics, 08/09/01, www.msnbc.com

Case 59

McGee, G. (2004) "Professor Hurlbut, Your 15 Minutes are Up," The American Journal of Bioethics Editors' Blog, 12/17/2004, http://blog.bioethics.net/2004/ 12/professor-hurlbut-your-15-minutes-are.html

Case 60

McGee, G. (2005) "Proposition 71 Has Created a Monster," The American Journal of Bioethics Editors' Blog, 01/10/2005, http://blog.bioethics.net/2005/01/proposition-71-has-created-monster.html

Conclusion

McGee, G. (2007) "A Hot and Cold Running Genius," *The Scientist,* 21(1): 24

McGee, G and Caplan, A. (2005) "Science Must Slow its Speed," Albany Times-Union, 12/15/2005

Index

Bioethics for Beginners: 60 Cases and Cautions from the Moral Frontier of Healthcare,
First Edition. Glenn McGee.
© 2012 John Wiley & Sons, Ltd. Published 2012 by John Wiley & Sons, Ltd.